THE ALLERGY BOOK

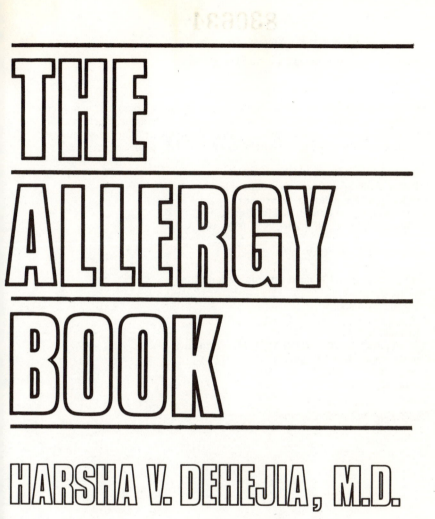

THE ALLERGY BOOK

HARSHA V. DEHEJIA, M.D.

 VAN NOSTRAND REINHOLD COMPANY
NEW YORK   CINCINNATI   TORONTO   LONDON   MELBOURNE

Copyright © 1981 by Personal Library, Toronto
Library of Congress Catalog Card Number 80-28336

Printed and bound in Canada
A Personal Library publication produced for
Van Nostrand Reinhold Company
A division of Litton Educational Publishing, Inc.
135 West 50th Street, New York, NY 10020, U.S.A.

16 15 14 13 12 11 10 9 8 7 6 5 4 3 2 1

Library of Congress Cataloging in Publication Data
Dehejia, Harsha V.
  The allergy book.

  Includes index.
  1. Allergy. I. Title [DNLM: 1. Hypersensitivity
Popular works. WD 300 D322a]
RC584.D4   616.97   80-28336
ISBN 0-442-21887-7

Printed and bound in Canada

Dedicated to all my patients from whose questions and concerns this book has arisen and to Lazarus J. Loeb, M.D., who sparked my interest in Allergy.

TABLE OF CONTENTS

PREFACE

Allergy is one disease which is reversible if well-managed. A patient can learn what is causing his reactions, can learn how to eliminate it from his environment, and with the help of his physician, can learn which treatment works best. Therefore it is absolutely vital to have a good reliable source of information such as this about allergy, what triggers it, and what can be done to relieve it.

Although I did not realize it at the time, Christmas Eve 1964 was a turning point in my life. My baby daughter culminated months of ill-health and ill-temper by going into shock when given a sip of egg-nog. A frantic trip to the hospital emergency ward resulted in the diagnosis of acute food allergy and asthma. Several more frightening trips to the hospital convinced me that I had better learn all I could about this enemy of my daughter's well-being — allergy.

Misinformation abounded when I began my search for knowledge. There was the dietitian who advised me to use a certain brand of cheese as it was milk-free; and the young intern who told me that "no one ever died of asthma." In the sixteen years that I have spent collecting information about allergy not only for my own family, but the families of thousands of allergic Canadians, I have become even more dedicated to the concept that to know allergy is to conquer it.

Since my involvement in 1964 with allergy there have been dramatic swings in theory: from the 'poor mothering' and 'emotional maladjustment' belief, so prevalent when my daughter was experiencing her problems, to the other extreme, that allergy was the cause of virtually all illness. Now, a more balanced picture is emerging, and Dr. Dehejia is an able proponent of this sensible, sensitive viewpoint. With proper diagnosis and treatment a patient can be expected to respond favorably to his allergic condition.

There are still well-meaning people who will tell the allergic person or patient that "allergies are all in the head" or "if left alone allergy will disappear in a seven-year cycle" or "chihuahua will take the asthma from the patient." Information contained in *The Allergy Book* dispels such myths and replaces them with facts.

Allergy still possesses areas of mystery, not only for the layman but for much of the medical profession as well. Some facets of this disease are not thoroughly understood and some explanations still generate considerable controversy. But increasing interest in the field has created a growing body of literature of help to the patient. *The Allergy Book* is designed to bridge the gap in knowledge enabling allergy sufferers to receive the information they need in order to cope effectively.

Susan Daglish, President
Allergy Information Association
August, 1980

ACKNOWLEDGMENTS

Mrs. Sunny Phillips, Mrs. Louise Villeneuve and Mrs. Linda Labelle are nurses who, over the years, have not only helped me interpret the science of allergy but also have contributed immensely in developing the art of allergy as a specialty in my office. Mrs. Betty Davis and Mrs. Merilyn Woods have willingly typed and retyped the manuscript in addition to carrying the secretarial load of a busy practice. In Glenn Witmer I have found not only a publisher and friend but also a gardener who nurtures ideas like seeds so that they may blossom.

And finally my wife and my two boys, who are living examples of being able to cope with allergy: despite troublesome and sometimes disabling allergic symptoms they have never stopped participating in the beauty and wonder of life, inspiring and encouraging me to write.

H.V. Dehejia, M.D.

PROLOGUE

Reading a book on allergy does not enable you to cope with allergies any more than a road map will take you to your destination. Both will help you in getting ready for the journey and will guide you along the route and prevent you from making false turns or taking a bumpy road. Perhaps after you reach your destination and you put the map away you will doubt whether you needed the map after all, and one day many years later when you discover the dust-covered map among your papers it might remind you of the trip you took.

Forewarned is forearmed, for it is the unknown that evokes fear and anxiety. Allergy is mainly a conjectural art and it has almost no rules, but by observation and experience we have been able to develop some guidelines and principles. It is the purpose of this book to share this experience and observation with you. Some experiences are fairly uniform and can be laid down almost as dictum; others are rather personal and may vary from physician to physician; and some — those that are experimental or innovative — other physicians might dispute.

Every time I have spoken to patients, nurses, or doctors about allergic disorders or have attempted to answer their questions, I have left the meeting richer. It is the questions I could not answer that have taught me more. When I teach I learn at the same time. Writing this book has been a learning experience for me.

If it helps give you a better insight into allergies suffered by you or those for whom you love and care, if it encourages you to take allergies in your stride and cope with them rather than submit to them, if it helps you ask intelligent questions the next time you see your doctor, if it enables you to help others who are not avid readers like yourself, the purpose of the book is well served.

1

WHAT IS ALLERGY?

DEFINITION AND MECHANISMS

Every writer and every speaker should be allowed at least one gimmick or one funny line. Mine is about the two types of people. Many years ago, when I spoke about allergy I used to say: "There are two types of people — those who have allergies and those who will eventually get them!" In those days there were more skeptics than believers in allergy. About 5 years ago I changed that line to: "There are two kinds of people — those who have allergies and those who wish they had them!" For allergy seems to have become a fashionable disease, and I seem to spend more time convincing people that they do not have an allergy. This past year I have often begun my talks with the comment: "There are

19

two kinds of people — those who use inhalers and those who misuse them!''

WHAT EXACTLY IS ALLERGY?

A good definition of allergy is: ''A reaction to a harmless substance.'' The key word in this sentence is *harmless*. The substance capable of producing an allergic reaction is perfectly harmless to people at large but in even minute amounts can affect the person who is allergic to it. If you walk into an extremely dusty warehouse or a burning house it is normal for *anyone* to cough or choke or have sore eyes. This cannot be called an allergy, because dust from the warehouse or smoke from a burning house is not harmless. However, if from merely walking across your bedroom floor you sneeze several times, or if you break out in hives (urticaria) all over your body after eating only half a peanut, you probably have an allergy, because most people can walk across the bedroom floor or eat a peanut without any problems.

Now that you know what an allergic reaction is let us introduce the two basic terms used quite frequently in allergy. An allergen (also termed 'antigen') is any substance that causes an allergic reaction. An antibody is the substance your body produces in response to the antigen.

Is allergy commoner today than it was 20 years ago? Not really. There is a greater awareness of allergy on the part of both the patient and the doctor, so that allergic diseases are recognized. What used to be dismissed as just a summer cold is now probably recognized as hay fever. The only genuine increase is perhaps in drug allergy and contact allergy, mainly because there are so many more drugs and other potentially allergenic substances today than there were 20 years ago.

WHY DOESN'T EVERYBODY HAVE ALLERGIES?

Whether you will be an allergic person is determined genetically; that is, the tendency is inherited. Roughly 10 per cent of the members of any given population are potentially allergic; or, to put it another way, 10 per cent of any given population have the potential to produce antibodies in their system. (These people are also called atopic.) This does not mean that they will necessarily experience any allergic symptoms — they just may not. However, the other 90 per cent of the population never will experience an allergy. Unfortunately there are no simple tests at present to find out what kind of a person you are, allergy-prone or allergy-proof. Also, the exact genetic transmission of an allergy is not yet understood; therefore, although we can say that allergy runs in families, we cannot predict (unlike many other genetically determined diseases) how many members of a family are likely to suffer from allergy. Also, allergy can skip generations.

This type of allergy is called 'atopy'; that is, hereditary hypersensitivity to substances that are harmless to other people. Atopic diseases are caused by inhalants, foods, insects and drugs. (There is another type of allergic reaction, called 'delayed allergic reaction.' A good example of this is contact dermatitis, which is discussed in another chapter. Delayed allergic reactions are not genetic in origin and are not produced by antigen–antibody reactions in your system.)

THE MECHANISM OF ATOPIC REACTIONS

When an allergy-prone individual is exposed to an antigen, his body reacts by producing antibodies. When a sufficient number of antibodies have been produced, the

21

antigen combines with the antibody and this union liberates certain chemical compounds in the body. One of the most important substances is histamine. Histamine and other such substances are normal components of the body; under normal conditions, they are inside your body cells and perform a useful function. However, when an allergic reaction takes place, histamine leaves your cells and circulates in the body in excessive amounts. Histamine causes three basic responses: certain blood vessels constrict, certain others dilate, and this dilation causes leakage of fluid from the blood vessels into your tissues. All allergic reactions in any part of the body are caused by this basic response of histamine.

It is important to note that sufficient numbers of antibodies have to be produced before an allergic reaction takes place in the body. Therefore, an allergic reaction does not occur when a person is first exposed to the offending allergen — it is only on the second or repeated exposure that enough antibodies are produced. The interval between the body's exposure to the antigen and the development of allergic symptoms, which is called the latent period, is a characteristic feature of all allergic reactions. Understanding this latent period is very important. A very common question I am asked is: "I have had my dog (or cat) for 10 years. Why have I become allergic to it now?" The answer is that *because* you have had your pet so long you are allergic to it now — symptoms of allergy do not develop on your first contact with a dog or cat, and maybe not for several months or years afterwards. By the same token, a patient does not have an allergic reaction the first time he has penicillin; it is on the second or a subsequent exposure to penicillin that an allergic reaction may develop.

Although the onset of symptoms of an allergic reaction depends primarily on the presence of sufficient antibodies in your system, there are important secondary factors.

Therefore, a person with sufficient antibodies in his system may yet be devoid of allergy symptoms. These other factors that tip the allergy balance in the body so that symptoms develop are infection, stress and strain, hormonal changes, and diminished body resistance. Thus it is quite common for asthma to begin after a severe respiratory infection.

Thus, we can now define allergy as an abnormal reaction to a harmless substance in genetically predisposed individuals, caused by an antigen and antibody reaction and the resultant release of histamine.

THE NATURAL HISTORY OF ALLERGIC CONDITIONS

Once you have allergies, do you keep them for the rest of your life or do you outgrow them? Do allergy symptoms come in cycles?

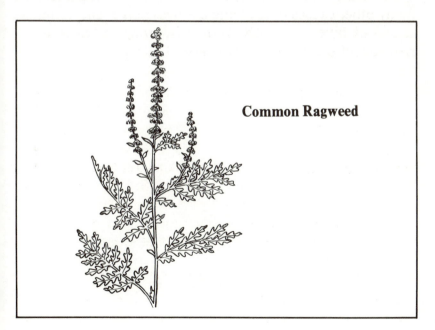

Common Ragweed

Because the tendency to allergies is inherited, if you are an allergic person you remain one all your life. This does not necessarily mean that you will have symptoms of allergy all your life, but your body will never lose its capacity to produce antibodies under the right conditions. Many people outgrow the symptoms of their allergy, but they never outgrow the allergic state. For example, hay fever may produce troublesome symptoms for a few years during childhood and then be quiescent for many years; this could be followed by asthma, which might last a few years and then again be followed by a lengthy quiescent period; and the same person, later on in life, could have an allergy to one or more drugs.

It is not true that allergy symptoms recur in any definite cycle or pattern.

Some common symptoms are sneezing, running eyes, rash, hives and wheezing. However, these and other allergy symptoms can be caused by other mechanisms, too: there are many other causes of sneezing besides allergy, and countless causes of hives or a rash. Thus it is wrong to regard every sneeze and every rash as evidence of allergy.

2

HAY FEVER

THE SUMMER COLD

Perhaps the commonest form of allergy is hay fever. The term 'hay fever' is really a misnomer, for the condition is neither caused by hay nor accompanied by fever, but like other misnomers the name will stay with us for a long time to come. Medically, the condition is called pollinosis or seasonal allergic rhinitis.

The manifestations of hay fever are runny eyes and nose, itchy eyes and nose, sneezing, red and swollen eyes, itchy palate and ears, and sometimes a rash. These symptoms can vary in severity from very mild, usually dismissed as just a summer cold, to very severe and distressing.

Hay fever is caused by pollens, which are the seeds of

flowers. But only certain pollens can cause hay fever: they must be microscopic in size and capable of being carried long distances by the wind. Pollens of common garden flowers such as marigolds and roses usually do not cause hay fever or allergies — such pollens are very large and sticky. The harmful pollens are those of trees, grasses, and weeds. All deciduous trees, such as maple, elm, poplar and birch, produce tiny flowers and blossom early in spring just before the leaves start growing. Likewise, grasses start growing in late spring and summer and produce tiny white flowers. (The blue-eyed grasses are actually members of the iris family.) Weeds bloom in the late summer. The weed most likely to cause hay fever is ragweed. Interestingly, ragweed grows only in North America.

Although cut flowers and garden flowers do not cause allergy, the wind can deposit on them pollens of trees, grasses, and weeds. This way, when these flowers are brought into the house, they can be an indirect source of trouble. The symptoms of hay fever are worse on a windy day and a dry day. Rain washes pollens away and therefore helps. Also, pollen is in its greatest concentration in the air in late evenings and early mornings. By and large the pollen count is higher in the countryside, but even large cities are not pollen-free. Obviously, activities such as cutting grass or working in the garden or playing in a field will increase your exposure to the harmful pollens.

No age is exempt from hay fever, but hay fever is usually a disease of the younger ages. The greatest incidence is between the ages of 5 and 35.

DIAGNOSIS

A proper history is the cornerstone in making a diagnosis of hay fever. Besides making a note of your symptoms,

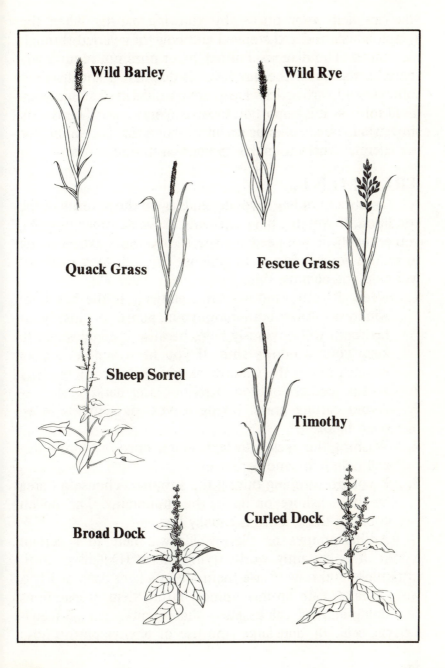

you can help your doctor by knowing exactly when the symptoms started and stopped and how they varied through the season. The diagnosis of hay fever does not require any special tests, but if the hay fever is distressing and troublesome — and particularly if you are considering having treatment for it — it is important to have allergy tests. These tests show what you are allergic to, information that is essential for the allergist who will make up your treatment serum.

TREATMENT

Treatment of hay fever depends upon the severity of the condition. If you just have sneezing in the summer months, you probably do not need any special treatment except trying to reduce your exposure to pollens. The following methods will help you achieve this.

1. Keep all your windows shut, particularly the bedroom windows. Air-conditioning your house or just your bedroom will obviously help, because it enables you to keep your windows shut. If you need ventilation, an exhaust fan in the window blowing outward helps.

2. Avoid needless outdoor activities after dark.

3. Avoid cutting grass, raking leaves, or activites in an open field.

4. Washing the eyes with tepid water once or twice a day will help itchy and sore eyes.

5. If you go camping during the summer, choose an area by the seashore or up in the mountains. The pollen count in these areas is usually low.

Antihistamines or allergy pills will help to a certain extent. It is certainly worth trying them. (Details of antihistamines and how to use them are in a later chapter.) It is wise to take plain antihistamines, rather than preparations containing antihistamines plus other agents such as acetylsalicylic acid. By and large, the use of phenylephrine nose drops and sprays is usually not recommended in allergic conditions. However, hay fever is perhaps an exception. If using a nose spray once at bedtime for a few days or weeks prevents sleepless nights, it is certainly well worth doing this, but long-term use of nose sprays is to be discouraged.

If your hay fever does not respond to these simple measures initiated by you, it is important to consult your doctor. Actually, even before you embark on treating your hay fever yourself, it is a good idea to check with your doctor and see if he approves of your plan. Hay fever that does not respond to simple measures, or whose symptoms are fairly distressing from the start, should be investigated properly. Your own doctor will probably examine you and perform allergy tests himself. (The tests are needed not only to find out what you are allergic to but also to determine the degree of your allergy.) However, your doctor may send you to an allergist or other specialist.

Having decided what specifically you are allergic to, and to what degree, the doctor will suggest the following measures.

1. Stronger antihistamines, if those you have already tried have not helped you.
2. Sodium cromoglycate by inhalation or Rynacrom intranasally.
3. Allergy injections (known as hyposensitization; that is, injections of minute but increasing doses of the allergic substances to increase your tolerance of them).

All three types of treatment can be taken singly or, better still, in combination.

UNTREATED HAY FEVER

Are there any consequences of leaving your hay fever untreated? One fact is certain: permanent damage will not result. However, once hay fever starts it is unlikely to go away for at least a couple of years, although the severity of your symptoms may vary from year to year depending on your body's resistance on the one hand and your exposure to pollens on the other. If, for instance, the summer is wet and you happen to spend most of your time indoors, your exposure to pollens will be greatly reduced and it is likely to be a good year for you.

Some of us believe that severe hay fever with chest symptoms such as cough or wheezing is likely to develop into bronchial asthma. Because of this and, more important, because allergy treatment of hay fever is so successful, I generally recommend that even moderately distressing hay fever be properly treated with a combination of environmental control measures, antihistamines, sodium cromoglycate, and allergy injections.

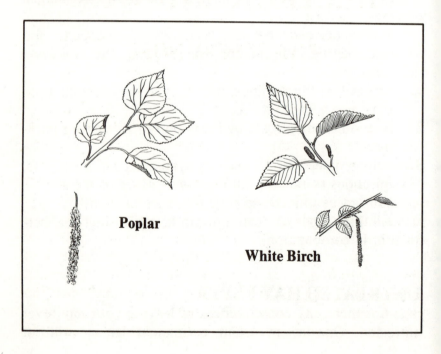

Poplar

White Birch

3

ALLERGIC RHINITIS

THE STUFFY NOSE

Allergic rhinitis — the stuffy-nose syndrome — is nasal stuffiness due to allergies. It results mostly from airborne allergens or inhalants.

As opposed to hay fever (whose symptoms are strictly seasonal), the stuffy-nose syndrome causes problems in any season or throughout the year. The symptoms are nasal stuffiness, sneezing, sniffing, runny nose, a postnasal drip (at the junction of the nose and the throat), and either lack of the ability to smell or an intolerance of smells. Sneezing and other nasal symptoms are worse in the morning when the patient is getting up and more severe indoors than outdoors. Also, these people are bothered by exposure to airborne pollutants (such as smoke), or sunlight, or to irritants such as water, chlorine or soap entering the nose.

If you have such symptoms you must proceed cautiously. In the first place, there are many other conditions that can mimic allergic rhinitis, and every stuffy nose is certainly not caused by an allergy. Secondly, there are very many allergens that can cause the stuffy nose — not just pollens, as in the case of hay fever. This condition is hard to self-diagnose, and it is even harder to self-treat. You must therefore seek medical help and let your doctor examine you.

Patients who have an allergic respiratory disease such as rhinitis or asthma are particularly intolerant of various airborne pollutants. It is important to distinguish pollutants from allergens (specific substances which produce harmful effects that cause an antigen–antibody reaction). Pollutants are nonspecific substances which, by their toxic or irritant nature, cause further inflammation of an already inflamed respiratory tract.

Although symptoms on exposure to pollutants and airborne allergens may be the same, it is important to differentiate between the two types of substances. For example, it is proper to say "I am intolerant of tobacco smoke" rather than "I am allergic to tobacco smoke." We are exposed to many pollutants in ordinary life, even in our own home. The commonest probably is tobacco smoke; following this are aerosols and sprays of all kinds, such as deodorants, hair-sprays, disinfectants, perfumes, window- and oven-cleaners, cleansers and polishes, plant-care products, lubricants, products for greaseless cooking, stain-removers, and waxes and other products for the care of household furniture.

Anything with a strong smell is also a pollutant for the allergic person; this includes, therefore, not only tobacco smoke but also cooking odors, paints and polishes, ammonia, and so on. Outside your home, also, you can be exposed to a large number of pollutants; these include automobile fumes, industrial pollution, sprays used on lawns and trees, and insect-repellents.

DIAGNOSIS

Whereas with hay fever a certain amount of self-diagnosis and self-treatment are permitted, with a stuffy nose that has persisted for some time and is troublesome you should make some pertinent observations about your symptoms and discuss the problem with your doctor. In making notes about this condition, you are well advised to pay attention to the following factors.

1. Even though your symptoms occur year round, are there any periods in the year when your symptoms are worse, and can you relate them to any special season or type of weather?
2. Are your symptoms less when you are indoors or outdoors?
3. Is there a sudden change in your symptoms from hour to hour?
4. What is the color of your nasal discharge? Is it thin and clear, or thick and colored?

There are some characteristic tell-tale signs of allergic rhinitis. Many people with allergies of the upper respiratory tract have bags and dark circles under the eyes; these result from congestion of the veins in and around the nose, and the appearance is sometimes referred to as 'allergic shiners.' Many patients, particularly children, who have allergic upper respiratory symptoms have a habit of rubbing their nose with the index finger or the whole hand. This is sometimes referred to as 'the allergic salute;' it seems to give them temporary relief by opening up the nasal passages, making it easier to breathe. This constant rubbing of the nose may lead to the development of a crease across the nose, which is called 'the allergic crease.' However, these superficial signs may not be present. In any event, a definite diagnosis of allergic rhinitis can be made only on examination of the nasal membranes, which is why you should consult your doctor. In allergic rhinitis, these membranes are characteristically bluish pink and examination of the nasal mucus under a microscope usually shows an abundance of a certain type of white blood cell, the eosinophil.

Allergy tests are required to confirm the diagnosis of allergic rhinitis and are absolutely essential if you are going to embark on allergy injections.

TREATMENT

Once allergic rhinitis has been diagnosed, the first step is to devise environmental control measures. Some *allergens* can be completely avoided and exposure to many can be reduced. Exposure to *pollutants and irritants*, also, must be reduced. The common inhalants are:

1. House dust, which includes substances such as feathers, wool, linen, cotton linters, cement and plaster, human hair and skin, and household insects.
2. Animal dander, which consists of minute scales from hair and skin, and saliva; bird (feather) dander.
3. Molds.
4. Miscellaneous: jute, kapok, pyrethrum (present in insecticides), glue, gum, orris root (in cosmetics), and newsprint.
5. Occupational dusts — which can be major factors for bakers, millers, woodworkers, etc.

Anyone with allergic rhinitis will be blowing his nose often. The patient is advised to use cloth handkerchiefs rather than tissues — cotton handkerchiefs are softer, and paper tissues can irritate the nose because of the fine paper-dust they generate and the chemicals they contain.

Allergy pills, which are a combination of an anti-histamine and a decongestant, help relieve the symptoms of allergic rhinitis. They must be taken regularly and a good time to take them is at bedtime. You may have to try a couple of varieties of allergy pills before you find the one that suits you best — some may cause drowsiness, and others make some patients hyperactive. If the allergy pill becomes ineffective because of the development of tolerance, your doctor will advise you to change the brand and try another variety. If one tablet at bedtime does not control symptoms throughout the day, you may need to take one in the morning or afternoon also. *Never use vasoconstrictive nose drops*: although they provide instantaneous, almost dramatic relief, their effect is short-lived and prolonged use of these drops damages the nasal membranes.

Allergy hyposensitization therapy has a definite place in the treatment of allergic rhinitis. These injections must be taken for at least 2 years and it is unusual to see any improvement in the first 4 to 6 months. If the rhinitis persists and all other forms of treatment have failed, cortisone may be needed. Cortisone can sometimes be injected into the nasal membranes. An alternative form is as a nasal spray. Cortisone nasal sprays must be used only under the supervision of your doctor, and their continuous and long-term use may be harmful. If a cortisone nasal spray is necessary, many doctors prescribe its use in 3-month cycles — the smallest effective dose for 2 months, then none for 1 month, and repeat the cycle.

4

VASOMOTOR RHINITIS

THE 'ALLERGY' THAT IS NOT AN ALLERGY

A 40-year-old woman complains of a constantly stuffy nose for the last 2 years. Her nose sometimes runs and occasionally she sneezes a lot. The stuffiness is perennial but at certain times it increases suddenly. Her symptoms are made worse by the smell of tobacco, detergents, and perfumes. She also has some headache.

If you listened to this story you would probably feel that this woman has indeed an allergy. Chances are that the woman who relates this story to her MD is convinced she has an allergy too. Yet the story is not that of an allergic stuffy nose. Obviously one needs to examine the patient and even do a few tests to make a diagnosis. Assuming that I examined the patient and did not find tell-tale signs of allergy in her nose and performed allergy tests that were all negative, I would make a diagnosis of vasomotor rhinitis.

Although this is not an allergy it masquerades as one. Therefore, let us discuss it in some detail.

In simple words, 'vasomotor rhinitis' means that there is an imbalance of circulation in the nose. And this is the basic disorder here: there is either too little or too much blood in the nose. Probably you have seen some people who have sweaty palms, or others who blush often and without reason, and are aware that some menopausal women get hot flushes. These are similar conditions and stem from similar mechanisms. Why this imbalance in circulation occurs is not clear. Sometimes it is hormonal in nature; even a slight imbalance of hormones in your body can cause this.

The condition not only causes nasal stuffiness but also leads to a very strong intolerance of smells. And many of these people carry a long list of smells they think they are allergic to (detergents, cleansers, waxes, perfumes, deodorants, tobacco, insecticides, industrial pollutants, and so on). These intolerances, of course, must not be regarded as a sign of allergy.

Well, how do you cope with this condition? First, accept the fact that this is not an allergy. This will prevent you from making the rounds of doctors' offices, from one specialist to another, seeking the elusive cause of this stuffy nose. Second, reduce environmental irritants. These include dust and strong smells.

The temptation to use nose drops to obtain relief is very great, and a large majority of these patients become very dependent on nose sprays and drops. The importance of avoiding nose sprays cannot be overemphasized: *nose sprays will not only stop working after a while but actually worsen the condition.*

37

Relief from nasal congestion should be sought from medications called decongestants, many of which are available over the counter in drug stores. Select a pure decongestant, rather than a combination product that also contains an antihistamine and an analgesic. Antihistamines have no place in the treatment of this condition, and analgesics do nothing for you unless you have an associated headache.

By and large the condition is mild and self-limiting and may last only a couple of years; when the imbalance of circulation is restored the condition corrects itself.

5

SINUSITIS

PAIN, POSTNASAL DRIP, AND POLYPS

Sinusitis (inflammation of the paranasal sinuses; i.e., of the sinuses in the region of the nose) is a specific disease of the upper respiratory tract, caused by a combination of allergy and infection. There is a tendency to use the word 'sinusitis' or simply 'sinus' to refer to any chronic nasal condition; this is inaccurate.

THE ANATOMY AND PHYSIOLOGY OF THE PARANASAL SINUSES

The paranasal sinuses are pairs of air sacs in your head and face. The largest of these is the maxillary sinus, which lies underneath the cheek bone. The frontal sinus is behind the eyebrows. And located deep in your head are the ethmoid and sphenoid sinuses. These sinuses communicate with the nose via small passages called ducts.

The paranasal sinuses perform several functions. First, they provide a reservoir of air in the upper respiratory tract. The air serves not only to balance any changes in pressure but also to warm and humidify the incoming air before it goes down into the lungs. Second, they have a very important function in giving your voice its special tonal qualities. Third, they reduce the weight of the head and face.

THE DUAL CAUSES OF SINUSITIS

Sinusitis (inflammation of the sinuses) is caused by two factors, allergy and infection. In some cases the predominant factor is allergy, in some others it is infection, and in many it is a combination of both. Since the nose and sinuses are in close proximity, the same allergens that affect the nose will affect the sinuses. These are therefore mainly the inhalants.

A third factor, which does not cause sinusitis on its own but is a major aggravating factor, is inhalation of pollutants or irritants.

Symptoms arise whenever there is a build-up of mucus in the sinus cavities and this mucus cannot drain into the nose because the duct is blocked. These symptoms include a sense of fullness in the head, facial pains particularly over one or both cheeks, headaches particularly above one or both eyebrows and on the forehead, nasal blockage and running, change in the voice, fever, a feeling of malaise and a postnasal drip.

Postnasal drip is the dripping of mucus and pus from the nose and sinuses into the back of the throat, and sometimes even into the respiratory tree. This causes symptoms such as throat-clearing, sore throats, a tickling sensation in the throat, episodic coughing (particularly at night), and wheezing. Occasionally, sinusitis causes only troublesome eye symptoms, such as pain in and behind the eyes, along with swelling of the upper and lower eyelids.

DIAGNOSIS

There are two phases of sinusitis, acute and chronic. In acute sinusitis, infection is the predominant factor. This condition lasts for a couple of days and clears up in response to a combination of antibiotics and decongestants. For only occasional episodes of acute sinusitis, one need not investigate the possibility of an allergic basis.

Chronic and recurrent sinusitis, however, needs investigation to discover whether it is due to allergy. This includes recording details of the history of your complaint and proper examination of your nose and upper respiratory tract. Microscopic examination of nasal mucus is a helpful test. An x-ray film of the sinuses is absolutely essential because there are many sinuses behind the nose and eyes that cannot be examined in the doctor's office. Skin tests will help in revealing the underlying allergy.

TREATMENT

The treatment of chronic recurrent sinusitis must be aimed at the underlying allergy, eradicating the associated infection, and preventing exposure to pollutants and irritants that could exacerbate the inflammation.

Treatment of the underlying allergic condition consists in avoiding the offending allergen and, in many cases, undergoing allergy hyposensitization therapy. As a build-up of mucus in the nose and paranasal sinuses is a major feature of chronic recurrent sinusitis, antihistamines and decongestants are an important part of treatment. Most of the pills advertised for treating sinusitis contain a combination of

41

antihistamine, decongestant, and analgesic, but if you have little or no pain it is better to choose a brand that contains no analgesic. You should take the medication regularly; a good time to take it is at bedtime. If the medication seems to lose its effect after a little while, change to another of the many available antihistamine/decongestant preparations.

The infective component of sinusitis needs treatment with appropriate antibiotics, which may have to be continued for several weeks before the infection clears completely. In certain circumstances, infections may have to be anticipated; this is why your doctor may prescribe antibiotics even if infection is minimal or absent. (Giving drugs to *prevent* infections is called chemoprophylaxis.) Determining which antibiotic will be appropriate may require laboratory culture of the nasal mucus to identify the germ and determine its sensitivity to various antibiotics.

Certain old-fashioned remedies for the relief of chronic sinusitis, such as inhaling steam or applying hot packs, cannot be dismissed altogether; they help to thin the nasal mucus and encourage drainage of clogged sinuses. It is sometimes better to alternate inhalation of steam with the application of ice-packs to the face.

If night-time cough due to postnasal drip is a troublesome feature of chronic recurrent sinusitis, the addition of a cough-suppressant to the antihistamine at bedtime will help. Also, raise the head of the bed (use an extra pillow, or put blocks under the top end of the bed); this will reduce the postnasal drip. For intractable sinusitis, when the infection has become lodged in the sinuses and recurrent courses of antibiotics and anti-allergy treatment have not helped, surgical drainage of the sinuses may become necessary. However, the need for sinus surgery has decreased in recent years, chiefly because of the better anti-allergy treatments and the wider range and greater potency of antibiotics.

Swimming should be avoided because it is especially troublesome to people who have sinusitis. This is not because of the exposure to chlorine (although this does irritate the nasal membranes): water entering the nose and the sinus cavities seems to churn the mucus and pus within them. Thus, swimming may exacerbate all the usual symptoms of sinusitis and even, in some people, cause coughing and wheezing for several days afterward.

NASAL POLYPS COMPLICATING SINUSITIS

Nasal polyposis (the formation of polyps in the nose) is an extension of sinusitis. In some people, when the infection is chronic and resistant the lining of the sinuses (the mucosa) becomes waterlogged and forms small grape-like projections; these are called polyps. The polyps may be completely within the sinuses or they may extend via the duct into the nasal cavity and occupy the back of the nose.

The symptoms of nasal polyposis are not very different from those of sinusitis. Likewise, its treatment is the same, at least in the majority of cases. The only difference is that if the polyps do not respond to one or two courses of antibiotics and antihistamines, it is preferable to have them surgically removed (polypectomy). Some nasal polyps can be removed under local anesthesia in an outpatient setting, but in certain cases admission to hospital is necessary.

One interesting feature of nasal polyposis is that some patients with this condition are allergic to ASA (the generic name is acetylsalicylic acid, usually abbreviated to ASA; trade names include Aspirin and A.S.A.). Not everybody with nasal polyposis need avoid ASA, but I recommend that they be careful with it and watch out for signs of ASA allergy.

Nasal polyposis may precede or accompany bronchial asthma.

SEROUS OTITIS

Serous otitis is a condition of the middle ear caused by an accumulation of serous fluid in the middle ear cavity leading to symptoms such as earaches and deafness. It is more common in younger children than adults and is very often associated with a nasal allergic condition.

Treatment of serous otitis is directed mainly towards the treatment of the associated nasal allergy. However, if there is no improvement, the fluid from the middle ear has to be drained and a tiny tube may be inserted for several months to drain this fluid continuously. Fortunately the condition does not result in long-lasting side effects.

6

BRONCHIAL ASTHMA

ALL ABOUT WHEEZING

WHAT IS ASTHMA?

Bronchial asthma can be defined as a condition characterized by recurrent but reversible episodes of wheezing. This definition implies two features. First, the wheezing has to be recurrent: a few isolated episodes that occur in various circumstances and in relation to different conditions do not constitute bronchial asthma. Second, the wheezing has to be reversible: there must be symptom-free intervals between episodes. (Continual wheezing is more likely to indicate bronchitis or emphysema.) Thus the diagnosis of asthma requires repeated observation and cannot be made at the first sign of wheezing.

MECHANISMS OF ASTHMA

Asthma is essentially a disease of the larger and medium-sized air passages, the bronchi; the smaller air passages (bronchioles) and the air sacs of the lungs are usually not involved. Normally, healthy bronchi are soft and kept widely open and their lining membrane is a healthy pink; they contain some mucus, which is kept in constant motion by minute hair-like processes called cilia. The movement of air in and out of normal lungs is a very smooth, effortless, noiseless process. In an asthmatic person, however, the bronchi are irritable and go into a state of spasm under certain conditions; the lining membranes are inflamed and swollen, and the amount of mucus within the respiratory tree (see A Dictionary For the Allergic, Chapter 18) may be increased. The bronchial spasm and the swelling (which reduces the lumen, the inside diameter of the bronchial passages), combined with the excess of mucus, obstruct air flow through the respiratory tract. Normally, inspiration (drawing air into the lungs) is fairly passive, as air is sucked in mainly due to the negative pressure in the chest. Expiration is an active process, however, and needs the bellows-type action of the chest wall and diaphragm to push the air out. This is why wheezing in bronchial asthma is mainly expiratory.

CAUSES OF ASTHMA

What makes the bronchi of the asthmatic different from those of others? We can talk at length about this and yet not answer that question — in fact, we don't know the full answer. Genetic factors are obviously important as asthma tends to run in families. Perhaps asthmatic people inherit a

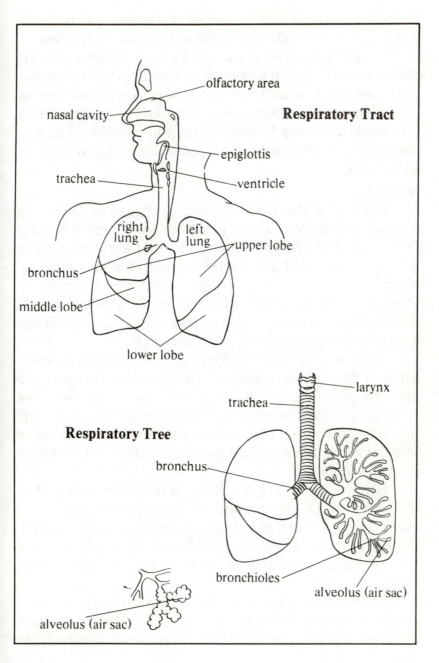

olfactory area

nasal cavity

Respiratory Tract

epiglottis

trachea

ventricle

right lung

left lung

upper lobe

bronchus

middle lobe

lower lobe

larynx

trachea

Respiratory Tree

bronchus

bronchioles

alveolus (air sac)

alveolus (air sac)

deficiency of certain nerve cells in the bronchi, a condition that could make them vulnerable to episodic obstruction.

In such people, who are said to have 'abnormal bronchial reactivity' (irritable bronchi), what are the factors that trigger an attack of asthma? These triggering factors can be divided into two broad groups, primary and secondary. There are only two primary factors, allergy and infection. The secondary factors are three: activity, emotion, and environmental irritants.

Allergy

Allergy is the most important triggering factor. In younger asthmatics, allergy is almost always the dominant factor. Inhalant allergy (allergy to inhaled allergens such as dust, pollens, mold and dander) is the predominant type; allergy to foods or drugs is less commonly the cause of asthma. Nearly all patients whose asthma is wholly or chiefly allergic have a history of one or more atopic manifestations such as eczema, hay fever, or food allergy.

Asthma brought on by allergy to pollens or molds is seasonal; it follows the season of the offending allergens and may be accompanied by hay-fever-type symptoms. The symptoms usually develop during the late evening and early morning and relate to activities like walking in areas of vegetation, gardening or cutting grass, or after visits to barns, farms, or stables.

Asthma due to dander allergy is obviously worse when the patient is in the company of the offending animal. A characteristic feature of asthma due to this cause is worsening of the wheezing in the middle of the night, probably because the concentration of dog or cat hair is highest at that time.

Bronchial asthma is rarely due exclusively to food allergy — inhalant allergies, also, are present in most cases. Theoretically, one can be allergic to just about any food, but

48

common allergenic foods are milk, eggs, fish (especially shellfish), cereals, nuts and seeds. Food allergy is dealt with in a later chapter.

Infection

Respiratory infection, the other primary triggering factor, is the second-commonest cause of bronchial asthma. The infection can be anywhere in the respiratory tract, from the nose down into the lungs. We do not know whether it is the germs themselves or their breakdown products that are responsible for the asthma. Viral infections are more likely than bacterial ones to precipitate an attack; what very often is a common cold 'goes to the chest' and causes cough and wheezing. Another source of respiratory infection is chronic sinusitis: the chronically infected sinuses contain a pool of mucus, which is readily infected, and the infected mucus drips down into the lower respiratory tract.

Activity

Activity is a major secondary triggering factor. Exercise tolerance varies greatly from patient to patient: some asthmatics can tolerate unlimited activity, whereas others may wheeze on even the slightest exertion. Furthermore, some asthmatics who wheeze only on exertion do not seem to have the underlying primary factors (allergy and infection).

The exact mechanism of exercise-induced wheezing is not known but most probably the reaction is mediated through the cells of nerves that govern one's breathing. Certain activities, like jogging, hockey, and downhill skiing, are more apt to produce wheezing than those like swimming, walking, and golf. In general, noncompetitive activities and sports are better tolerated. Activity combined with exposure to cold air can be particularly troublesome to the asthmatic.

Emotion

It is very difficult to make any definite statement about the role of emotion in any disease and particularly so in a condition like asthma. Medical opinion can vary between two extremes, with every shade in between: some doctors, particularly psychiatrists, insist that asthma is a wholly emotional problem, whereas others consider emotion a negligible factor. In fact, it is rather rare for asthma to be caused entirely by emotional factors but quite common for emotion to be a major secondary triggering factor — many asthmatics have more symptoms when under stress at home, school, or work.

Do asthmatics have a certain kind of personality? I do not think so. Cause should not be confused with effect: although the role of emotional factors in the *cause* of asthma is debatable, there is no doubt that chronic troublesome asthma can give rise to emotional problems such as anxiety, frustration, depression, and loss of self-image.

Environmental Irritants

Asthmatics are particularly sensitive (not allergic) to the quality of the air they breathe, and any variation in this may trigger symptoms of asthma. The quality of air is influenced by factors such as temperature and humidity, and its composition is altered by environmental irritants and pollutants such as automobile exhaust fumes, industrial pollutants, smoke, aerosols and sprays, and substances with a strong aroma such as paints, polishes, perfumes and cooking odors.

SYMPTOMS OF ASTHMA

The principal symptom of asthma is recurrent wheezing. This may be very occasional or fairly frequent and can be induced by a combination of primary and secondary factors. It is difficult to define precisely an episode of asthma as such, as individual tolerance of wheezing varies considerably. The first experience of slight wheezing can be quite frightening, whereas patients who wheeze often learn to live with this daily. Also, under some conditions an asthmatic may have only cough and no wheezing. Therefore, what is an attack of asthma for one may not be for another.

Despite this variation in the degree of tolerance to wheezing, certain symptoms and signs must be taken to indicate very severe asthma. They are:

1. Retraction (indrawing) of the muscles around the neck and the ribs.
2. Cyanosis (blueness) of the lips and nail-beds.
3. Alteration of mentation, like drowziness and somnolence.

The last two symptoms suggest severe, and even grave, asthma.

The late evening and early morning are particularly troublesome for the asthmatic. There are several reasons for this. First, lying down is not an ideal position for asthmatics — they breathe best when sitting up. Second, mucus tends to accumulate when one is sleeping, because of a combination of mechanical factors and the diminished movement of the cilia (hair-like processes in the bronchi). Third, the concentration of cortisone in the body drops at night, and this causes the bronchi to be more irritable.

A word about wheezing. The degree of loudness of wheezing depends upon the site of its production: loud wheezing is produced in the upper air passages, whereas wheezing that is inaudible or is detectable only by putting one's ear to the patient's chest is produced in the smaller air passages. It is important to realize that, even after disappearance of an audible wheeze, the smaller bronchi may remain constricted for as long as 48 to 96 hours.

If you have asthma, make a note of the conditions or factors that bring on wheezing. This will not only help you to anticipate wheezing — and thereby avoid or minimize it —

but will also help the doctor in making the proper diagnosis.

NATURAL HISTORY OF ASTHMA

"How long shall I wheeze?" or "When will my child outgrow his asthma?" is a very common and reasonable question, but it is difficult to answer with any degree of precision.

The following factors augur a better future for the patient. First, age at onset: the outlook is brighter for patients who are neither very young (less than 1 year of age) nor too old (over 40 years). Second, the patient who has purely allergic asthma tends to do better than the one who has purely intrinsic (infective-type) asthma. Third, the asthmatic who wheezes only sporadically has a better future than one who wheezes continuously. Fourth, the asthmatic who responds to even small amounts of bronchodilators has a better chance of outgrowing his asthma than one who needs various medications, admissions to hospital, or prolonged cortisone therapy.

TREATMENT

When considering the treatment of any allergic disease, and asthma in particular, one should always pay more attention to preventive measures than to the treatment of symptoms. There are several things you can do to prevent asthma attacks or reduce their severity and frequency.

Preventive Measures

First, a proper understanding of the disease, particularly the triggering factors, is absolutely essential: once you know what precipitates your asthma, you can take steps to avoid those situations or factors or, if that is not possible, you can anticipate the symptoms and be prepared to cope with them. These steps include environmental control, avoidance of pollutants and irritants, prompt recognition and treatment of respiratory infections, and regulation of activity to suit your tolerance.

Second, allergy injections (desensitization therapy) help reduce the effects of predisposing allergic factors. But remember, this therapy will not help the person who has intrinsic asthma, where infection is the major problem.

Third, sodium cromoglycate (Intal) is a true preventive medication and works well for the asthmatic in whom the allergic factor is predominant. This drug must be taken before the patient comes in contact with the allergen and throughout his exposure to it; for example, an asthmatic who wheezes only on exposure to ragweed must start using Intal 1 week before the ragweed pollinates and continue it until at least 1 to 2 weeks after the first frost. Occasionally, Intal also helps prevent asthma brought on by exposure to cold air or after activity.

Fourth, bronchodilators taken before the onset of asthma may prevent wheezing. For example:

1. The asthmatic who wheezes because of recurrent respiratory infections would be better off if he took a bronchodilator at the first sign of infection.
2. The child who wheezes during a hockey game would do better if he took medication before the game.

Bronchodilator Drugs (see Chapter 15 also)

The symptomatic treatment of asthma revolves around the intelligent and proper use of bronchodilators. There are two main types, the aminophylline group and the *beta*-2-stimulator group; you can use either one or combine the two, but you must depend upon your own doctor to prescribe the single bronchodilator or combination that is best for you.

These drugs can be taken by various routes — by mouth (orally), inserted into the rectum, by inhalation, or intravenously. The oral route is to be preferred at all times. Bronchodilators taken orally start to work within 30 minutes and their action lasts about 4 to 6 hours; therefore, the medication should be repeated every 4 to 6 hours during the day. When wheezing is severe and troublesome, the treatment should be continued around the clock, night and day. Also, anyone who wheezes more than twice a week should take the drug continually rather than sporadically. Finally, bronchodilators must be continued for at least 48 to 96 hours after audible wheezing has ceased.

Hand-held bronchodilator inhalers (nebulizers) provide instant relief and have reduced the need for injections of epinephrine and visits to hospital emergency departments. However, it is important to understand some of the shortcomings of this therapy. First, the relief it provides is instant but short-lived. Second, to provide maximal benefit the inhaler must be held properly and the medication must be released at the right time so that it enters your respiratory system and is not lost outside your mouth. Third, absorption of the medication (and perhaps even the propellant) into your system is thought to be responsible for some serious cardiac side-effects.

There are only two indications for using a nebulizer: to abort a sudden, unexpected bout of cough or wheezing in someone who is already taking bronchodilators orally; and when it is very inconvenient to take tablets (such as in an arena, in some situations at school or in an office, or during the night). If used sparingly and intelligently, a nebulizer can be very useful. If you find you are using the inhaler 4 or more times a day, you should consult your doctor immediately.

Emetics, or Drugs that Induce Vomiting

This is an old-fashioned remedy for breaking an attack of asthma. The drug that is commonly used is called ipecac. The exact mechanism of the action is not known, but many asthmatic children feel better after vomiting.

Cortisone

The 'wonder drug' cortisone does wonders for asthma, too. It helps the asthmatic by reducing inflammation within the bronchi, suppressing the allergic reaction, and causing the bronchi to dilate. However, prolonged use of cortisone can produce serious and disabling side-effects; therefore, cortisone should be used only under supervision of a doctor and as little as possible.

There are only two indications for cortisone: to relieve a severe acute exacerbation of chronic asthma, and to treat intractable chronic asthma that has not responded to bronchodilators. For acute exacerbations of chronic asthma, cortisone pills will bring about relief in 48 to 96 hours. Once wheezing has subsided, cortisone should be discontinued over the next 3 or 4 days. Some doctors recommend stopping the cortisone abruptly whereas others prefer tapering it off. Such 'bursts of cortisone' have no appreciable side effects and have changed the lives of many who previously had severe, disabling asthma.

Physical Therapy

Breathing exercises, yoga, swimming and other forms of physical conditioning, performed individually or in a group, are beneficial. They not only improve the asthmatic's self-confidence and morale but also, under certain conditions, may reduce wheezing by improving the tone of the nerves that are concerned in your breathing mechanism.

A person who has learned the art of relaxed expiration is able to perform better and to withstand the stresses of an acute episode of asthma. Just as a car performs best when properly tuned, a person is best able to enjoy life and cope with problems when in best possible condition.

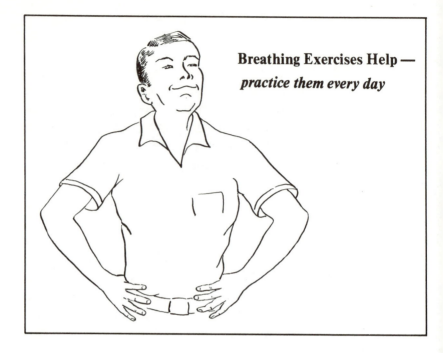

Breathing Exercises Help —
practice them every day

'FARMER'S LUNG'

Farmer's lung, also called extrinsic allergic alveolitis, is an allergic condition of the lung caused by inhalation of moldy hay dust. Obviously farmers are the most frequent candidates but anyone exposed to the offending mold can contract the disease. Disease states similar to, if not identical with farmer's lung, can occur in workers engaged in other occupations. These include pigeon breeders, individuals who are exposed to the compost used for growing mushrooms, and workers exposed to the dust generated from moist bagasse (the cellulose fiber of sugar cane), stripping the bark off maple trees, or exposed to moldy malt or barley dust.

When hay that is taken into storage is damp it gets moldy. When bales of hay that have become moldy are opened the mold spores are released as a white powdery dust. In allergy-prone persons, inhalation of this dust in sufficient amounts causes symptoms such as cough, congestion, expectoration, shortness of breath and wheezing. In the initial stages the condition may resemble an episode of influenza, with symptoms such as fever and malaise. Unlike bronchial asthma, farmer's lung produces scars in the lung and leads to progressive deterioration in lung function.

Farmer's lung is a disease which tends to be overlooked and the diagnosis is very often missed. A high index of suspicion is most important. Allergy skin tests may not help very much. The finding of a specific precipitin in the blood is diagnostic of this condition. Farmer's lung, unlike bronchial asthma, responds poorly to bronchodilators; the medication of choice is cortisone.

It is important on the one hand not to equate farmer's lung with bronchial asthma, although the symptoms may be similar, and on the other hand not to confuse it with silo-filler's disease, which is a type of chemical pneumonia caused by inhalation of the noxious fumes that accumulate in farm silos.

7

CROUP

'WHEEZING', YET NOT AN ALLERGY

Croup, medically called tracheobronchitis or laryngotracheobronchitis (depending on the extent of the disease), masquerades as an allergy and therefore is discussed in this book. First, its symptoms are rather similar to those of asthma; they consist of cough, choking, stridor (which sounds something like wheezing) and drooling. (Stridor is low-pitched and occurs during inspiration, whereas wheezing is high-pitched and occurs during expiration.) Second, the symptoms are recurrent. Third, they are made worse by factors such as activity and exercise and exposure to irritants.

Croup is an infectious process and not an allergy. It occurs in infants and young children. Most of these children experience only an isolated episode and recover from it rather nicely, but if the symptoms do not respond to simple measures (see below) you should take the child to the nearest hospital emergency department. However, some children have a croup-like illness several times a year. It is hard to say whether they get different infections or the same infection persists, but it is important not to regard this as an allergy and certainly not an allergy 'to their own germs.' Perhaps these children with recurrent croup have an altered immunity which makes them more susceptible to infections and, at the same time, some deficiency in their bronchial wall that causes them to hyperreact to stimuli such as infections and irritants.

The frustration and concern of the parents of such croupy children are genuine. An attack of croup is most unpleasant, and many of these parents go from doctor to doctor looking for the elusive cause.

The management of croup consists of three things — humidity, bronchodilators, and antibiotics. Humidity can be provided by a bedside humidifier or, in the acute stages, by holding the child in your arms just beyond the spray from a very warm shower. Bronchodilators usually give short-term relief. Antibiotics may have to be given recurrently and often for long periods.

The future for these croupy children is very bright. They grow out of this chronic condition into normal healthy children, and there is no reason to believe that in later life they will have asthma, bronchitis, or emphysema.

8

ALLERGIC ECZEMA

ITCH AND SCRATCH

Allergic eczema, also called atopic dermatitis, is a skin disorder characterized by dryness and itching. Some people call every skin problem 'eczema' and regard every rash as an allergic rash, but atopic (allergic) eczema is a specific disease with definite signs and symptoms.

The basic abnormality is not, surprisingly, an underlying allergy, but a congenital deficiency of sweat glands. Normally, sweat glands produce a thin film of moisture on the skin; this is called invisible sweating. Deficiency in this 'invisible sweat' causes dryness. Although it is not caused by an allergy, in many cases this type of eczema is associated with an allergic tendency and may precede allergic manifestations such as hay fever.

60

There are two types of allergic eczema, the infantile type and the childhood/adult type. Infantile eczema begins in the first year, very often in the first week of life. The childhood/adult type begins most often before puberty. In infantile eczema, there is a strong association with allergy to foods such as milk, cereals, eggs, citrus fruits and vegetables. In the childhood/adult type, however, this association with allergy to foods is less evident, and unless the skin condition definitely worsens in relation to certain foods no attempt should be made to investigate for allergies.

The skin lesions have a characteristic appearance and location. The affected skin appears dry and cracked. The patches are most commonly in the creases of the body, such as those of the wrist and forearm, face, neck, around the eyes and ears, behind the knees and on the legs. The predominant symptom is itching, which leads to scratching, and this in turn causes more itching (the scratch/itch cycle); this causes redness of the skin. The eczema can vary from very mild to very severe. If the eczema is severe and widespread, involving large areas of the body, the lesions may swell and ooze and the patient's hair (including eyebrows) may fall out.

DIAGNOSIS

Allergy tests are not necessary to establish the diagnosis of allergic eczema. However, they may be helpful in the infantile type — although a food diary is more useful, and possibly a trial elimination of certain foods.

TREATMENT

The main treatment is directed toward maintaining the skin's natural moisture and avoiding irritation. Emollients (creams, oils, and ointments) help to retain the natural moisture; they should be bland, nonperfumed, and non-medicated. A good time to apply these agents is after a shower or bath, so that the newly acquired moisture is held on. For troublesome eczema on the arms or legs, wrapping plastic around the part after applying cream or ointment helps to retain the emollient longer. The best time to do this is at bedtime.

Paradoxically, baths and showers, although they give short-term relief from itching, reduce whatever moisture there is in the skin and in the long term increase the itching. Baths are worse than showers. Showers should be limited to one or two a week and the skin should be dabbed rather than rubbed. Finger- and toenails should be clipped short; it may be necessary to cover an infant's hands, particularly if he tends to scratch at night. Clothes next to the skin should be of cotton; thus, underclothes, nightclothes, and bedlinen should not contain wool or flannelette.

Antihistamines (taken orally) help to reduce the itching. It is a good idea to have a dose at bedtime, to ensure a good night's sleep. If inflammation of the skin is a problem, cortisone creams and ointments will help. These must be applied on the affected areas and if necessary covered with a plastic wrap. Cortisone is absorbed to a certain extent, even through the skin, and therefore should be used as sparingly as possible.

Frequent scratching leads to infection in the skin; this takes the form of a yellow discharge or pustules. Whenever there is an infection complicating atopic eczema, this should be treated with antibiotics orally and not antibiotic creams.

Smallpox vaccination must not be performed on a patient who has allergic eczema.

Severe atopic eczema can be a very frustrating condition for both parent and child, and you will need a fund of patience and perseverance to overcome it.

9

CONTACT DERMATITIS

THE ALLERGIC TOUCH!

A ring, a pair of shoes, a new shirt, hair dye and rubber! What do these harmless, mundane things have in common? Most of us come in contact with one or more of these items every day and suffer no ill effects, yet others break out in a rash. This is contact or allergic dermatitis. It differs from other kinds of allergic reactions in certain respects. First, prolonged and recurrent contact is essential to produce this reaction; occasional or sporadic contact is not enough. Second, the manifestations are essentially local and at the site of contact. Third, this kind of allergy is not mediated by the characteristic antigen–antibody reaction that occurs in hay fever or asthma. Contact allergy is not necessarily commoner in people who suffer from other types of allergy; the only exception perhaps is allergic eczema, where one might see an increased incidence of allergic dermatitis.

Any substance in sufficient amounts can cause contact dermatitis but certain substances are more capable of causing this than others. Contact dermatitis is also an occupational hazard.

Let us look at the question of contact dermatitis from two standpoints. First, let us focus our attention on the parts of the body and see how each part can be involved. Then let us consider each of the suspected agents.

Forehead	*Hatbands, hair dye*
Back of the neck and behind the ear	*Hair dye*
Eyelids	*Cosmetics of all kinds, including nail polish*
Ear lobes	*Earrings*
Face	*Cosmetics, razor*
Bridge of the nose	*Spectacles*
Nose and folds around the nose	*Nasal medications and cleansing tissue*
Lips	*Lipstick, toothpaste*
Neck	*Wool clothing, necklace*
Armpits	*Deodorant, clothing*
Hands	*Plants, household chemicals, detergents, occupational exposure, recreational chemical exposure, medications, cosmetics, rubber, metal*
Trunk	*Clothing, metal, and elastic*
Legs	*Clothing, objects carried in pockets*
Feet	*Stockings and shoes*

DIAGNOSIS

As the above list indicates, diagnosis is established by a high index of suspicion and a careful, almost detective-like history. In difficult cases and where the diagnosis is less obvious, patch testing may have to be carried out. This consists in applying a small amount of the material suspected of causing the allergy to the skin and covering it for about 24 to 48 hours. A positive test is seen as an area of redness and even hardness.

COSMETIC ALLERGY

Many patients are puzzled how they can become allergic to cosmetics they have been in contact with for years. "I haven't been using anything new" or "I haven't switched my brand of cosmetic," they will say, but this unfortunately is the nature of the beast. Because you have been exposing yourself to the substance for so many months or years you have now become allergic to it. If you did have a rash the first time you used a new cosmetic that would be an example of primary irritation and not allergic dermatitis. A doctor once remarked to me that he was overwhelmed by the number of patients with contact dermatitis due to cosmetics whom he saw in his practice. What overwhelms me, I said, is that we do not see more of it, when we consider the variety of cosmetics that men and women alike use these days. I feel we are getting away with it rather lightly!

Theoretically, any cosmetic can cause contact dermatitis, but some are more likely to than others. Hair dye is perhaps the worst offender. The offending agent in hair dyes is a chemical called paraphenylenediamine. The rash from hair-dye allergy appears typically behind the neck and ears and on the forehead. Shampoos, hair conditioners, rinses and tangle removers, also, can cause dermatitis. All manufacturers of hair dye recommend a test of the dye before you

65

start using it. This is done by applying a small amount of the dye either on the forearm or behind the ears and covering it with adhesive tape for about 24 hours. If the area becomes red within an hour or so this represents primary irritation — not an allergy. If it becomes red in about 24 hours this represents contact dermatitis. In either case, you should not use that hair dye. If, however, no reaction develops within 24 hours it means you are not already allergic to this dye — but it does not mean you will never have an allergic reaction to this dye. This last point is worth emphasizing.

Antiperspirants contain formaldehyde and aluminum salts, and deodorants contain neomycin, all very capable of producing contact dermatitis in the armpits.

Eye make-up (pencil, shadow, and mascara): all types can cause dermatitis of the eyelids.

Nail polishes contain formaldehyde and can cause dermatitis not only on the fingers but also on the eyelids.

Powders, creams, rouge, and aftershave lotions cause dermatitis because of the perfume they contain. Likewise, soaps also can cause dermatitis from the chemicals or perfume in them. (Note that many products are advertised as toilet or bath bars: they contain synthetic detergents and are not soap.)

When cosmetic allergy is suspected the following should be done. First, stop all cosmetics for at least 3 weeks, with the exception of lipstick and night cream and perhaps babies' shampoo. After all the rash has disappeared try to introduce only one cosmetic at a time per week. If you encounter the offending agent avoid it completely. Try a hypoallergenic brand if you must use that particular cosmetic (hypoallergenic brands are probably less harmful but not necessarily safe).

As a general rule, and this applies to both men and women, use as few cosmetics as infrequently as possible.

Clean your face with tepid water to wash away the cosmetic as soon as possible.

METAL DERMATITIS

The commonest form of metal dermatitis is that produced by nickel, chromium, or cobalt. These metals are found singly or in combination in just about any metallic object you come in contact with each day. Obviously, a rash from metal dermatitis will appear at the site of contact. The following is a partial list of metal objects that can cause contact dermatitis: jewelry, hairpins, hair rollers, eyelash curlers, razor, cigarette holder, mouthpiece of a musical instrument, watchband, furniture, zipper, button, buckle, belt and clips, scissors and silverware. Also, chromium salts are present in leather and in matchsticks.

As with the other allergies, the treatment of metal dermatitis is avoidance: avoid contact with metal as much as possible, particularly prolonged and recurrent contact. Therefore, articles such as buckles and belts that are likely to come in contact with your skin should be avoided or should be well padded with a fabric such as velvet. Jewelry should be made of gold, and inexpensive jewelry should be avoided.

Metal dermatitis can occur in relation to certain occupations, such as mining, photography (darkroom work), and automobile manufacturing.

CLOTHING DERMATITIS

Dermatitis resulting from contact with clothing is not due to the fabric but to the chemicals it contains. Clothing contains a large number of chemicals, such as dyes, size and other finishing agents, and substances that provide crease-resistance properties. Dermatitis due to clothing can occur on any part of the body but is commonest in the folds of the body and under tight-fitting clothing. Dermatitis of this type is commoner also in obese individuals and those who sweat more.

The following simple rules may prevent dermatitis due to clothing.

1. Do not wear an unwashed garment.
2. When clothes are returned from the cleaners, air them before wearing them.
3. Next to the skin, cotton is best. Also, do not wear colored undergarments.

PLANT DERMATITIS

This, also, is a fairly common form of contact dermatitis. It occurs particularly after contact with the *Rhus* family of plants, which includes poison ivy, poison oak, and poison sumac, and with hairy-leaved primula. This contact produces a very characteristic reaction, consisting of redness and water blisters, which can be local or fairly widespread. Some patients are so sensitive to these plants that actual contact with the plant is not needed and they can get the reaction even from the fumes of such plants being burnt in a campfire.

Again, avoidance is the best treatment. Patients with a known history of poison-ivy dermatitis should expose as little of their body as possible in the warmer months. They should be encouraged to wear gloves when working in the garden, and any such plants in their own backyard should be chemically destroyed.

Mild rashes can be treated with local creams and ointments, but any severe dermatitis has to be treated by your doctor with a short course of cortisone by mouth.

A form of desensitization therapy to these plants has been tried, but the results have been uniformly poor and therefore this treatment has been generally abandoned.

RUBBER DERMATITIS

Rubber is present in a wide variety of things, such as shoes, elastic, undergarments, gloves, furniture, adhesive tape and elastic bandages. It can produce a troublesome kind of dermatitis, particularly when the contact is prolonged and recurrent. Avoidance, once again, is the best treatment. When it comes to clothing, rubber should be either completely avoided or shielded by a fabric such as cotton or velvet. Paper tape may have to be used instead of the standard adhesive variety.

10

INSECT ALLERGY

LUMPS, BUMPS, AND EVEN SHOCK

All of you I am sure have been stung or bitten by an insect. The slight redness, swelling, pain and itch you experience is perfectly normal — it does not constitute an allergy. All insects have venom and this is a toxic chemical, and the degree of this normal or toxic reaction depends upon the amount and type of venom that was injected.

However, if you over-react to insect bites with the production of extremely large local reactions, a reaction that is unduly prolonged, or symptoms in other parts of the body, you probably have an allergy to that insect.

For the purposes of allergy these insects can be divided into two groups: the stinging insects and the biting insects.

THE BITING INSECTS

Let us consider the biting insects first. This group includes mosquitoes, sandfly, deerfly, horsefly, and so on. These insects produce what is called a delayed allergy; that is, the effects of the bite do not develop right away and may take several hours to appear. You are aware of the large, red, hard swellings that some people get after a mosquito bite. Swelling may involve the entire area around the bite, and even the glands in the armpit or groin. Sometimes this reaction is accompanied by fever, and the person can be quite sick. But the allergic reaction never goes beyond this — it is never dangerous or fatal. This is where it differs from allergy to stinging insects.

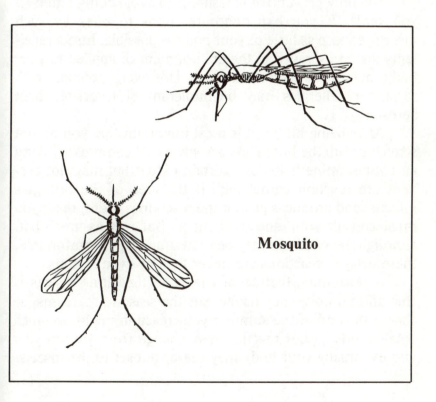

Mosquito

Treatment for Biting-insect Allergy

Contrary to popular belief there is no definite preventive treatment for allergic reactions to insect bites. In other words, no injections are available that would prevent the reactions to insect bites. Attempts to devise a program of allergy injections for mosquito bites have never been successful, partly because the allergic reaction is delayed (and not immediate, as in the case of stinging insects). A number of other preventive measures have been tried without any significant success. One that merits mention is the use of vitamin B_1 (thiamine) in large doses (200 mg. a day for adults), based on the claim that this prevents allergic reactions to mosquitoes by acting as a mosquito-repellant.

The only preventive measure is to avoid being bitten (if you can!). If you experience reactions to bites by such insects, expose as little of your body as possible. Insect repellents that are sprayed in the environment or applied to your body help to a certain extent. However, persons with respiratory allergies may be intolerant of insect-repellent aerosols.

After being bitten, it is most important that you do not scratch or rub the bitten area. Apply a cold compress. Taking an antihistamine helps to a certain extent but may not prevent the reaction completely. If the area of the bite gets infected and produces pus, or the reaction is widespread, you must consult your doctor about it. But rest assured that, although the swellings may be grotesque and uncomfortable, these delayed reactions are never fatal or even serious.

A redeeming feature of allergy to the biting insects is that an immunity may develop as the season progresses, so that at the end of the summer your reaction might be much smaller. Also, your reaction may change from year to year and eventually your body may cease to react to the insects.

THE STINGING INSECTS

The stinging insects are a class by themselves. In this group are included the bee, wasp, yellow-jacket and hornet. They produce what is called an immediate allergic reaction. In its simplest form there is a local redness and swelling; the next step is swelling of the entire area; and in its severe form it can cause generalized swelling, hives, choking, difficulty breathing, unconsciousness and even death. Thus, this kind of allergy is obviously more serious.

If you have ever manifested an allergic tendency, such as hay fever, eczema, or drug allergy, you are probably more vulnerable than others to insect allergy. Even without such a warning, however, your first experience with a bee sting can be quite alarming.

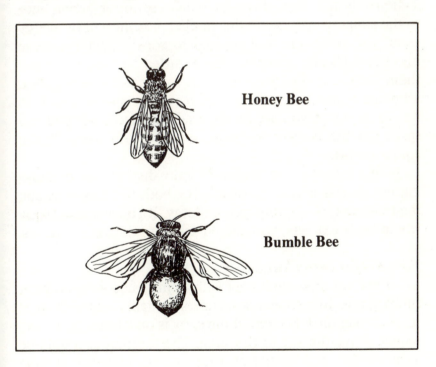

Honey Bee

Bumble Bee

Diagnosis of allergy to these insects is made principally by history. Tests of allergy to the stinging insects help not only in confirming the diagnosis but also in determining the degree of allergy.

Allergic reactions to the stinging insects should and could be prevented. In the first place, avoidance is the most important step. Expose as little of your body as possible. Do not invite trouble by disturbing a bees' or hornets' nest. Do not wear bright clothing or strong perfumes — these attract insects. When stung, do not panic — this only makes the situation worse and invites more insects.

There does exist a very effective program of hyposensitization injections for allergy to these insects. Only your doctor can decide whether you are a candidate for these injections. By and large, if you have had a serious reaction once to the stinging insects and this has been confirmed by allergy tests, you would be well advised to consider having these injections. Usually, once you have started on them you need them for the rest of your life, but fortunately the injection schedule is less demanding than for other allergies such as hay fever. Once you are on the maintenance dose, you can space out the booster injections every 4 to 6 weeks in the colder months.

Very recently, the venom of individual species of stinging insects has become available for both the diagnosis and the treatment of stinging-insect allergy. If you are now taking whole-body extracts, you should ask your doctor about this.

First Aid for Insect Stings

First, remove the stinger with a pin or needle — without rubbing it in (the stinger sometimes contains a good drop or so of the venom). Second, if the sting is on a limb, tie a tourniquet above the site of the sting. The tourniquet should be tight enough and should be kept on, but loosened slightly every 5 or 6 minutes for a few seconds, for at least 30 minutes, then loosened for another 30 minutes. Apply an icepack to the area of the sting, and take an antihistamine or an allergy pill as soon as possible.

Severe reactions

If you have had a violent reaction in the past, or if your doctor considers you are very sensitive to these insects, it is wise to carry a syringe containing an epinephrine solution. This is available in drug stores singly or in a kit. If a serious reaction such as choking develops, it is imperative that you have an injection of epinephrine right away (if this is self-administered, a good area is the outer side of the thigh) — go to the nearest doctor or hospital emergency department without wasting any time.

Patients with known heart disease should check with their doctors before using epinephrine.

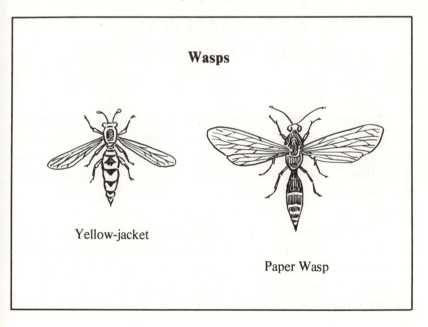

Wasps

Yellow-jacket

Paper Wasp

11

FOOD ALLERGY

ONE MAN'S FOOD,
ANOTHER MAN'S POISON!

It is not surprising that, with something so essential to human life as food, man has attributed to food everything from eternity to disease. It has been proclaimed since antiquity that "you are what you eat," and yet equally rightly it has been said that "one man's food is another man's poison."

Foods can cause problems in many ways. First, there can be dislike or even aversion to food purely because of psychological reasons. Second, food can cause difficulties by merely physical factors; for example, spicy food can cause heartburn, and a heavy meal may result in discomfort. Third, foods are maldigested or malabsorbed in patients with certain disorders; for example, milk is not absorbed in lactase deficiency, cereals containing gluten cannot be digested in cystic fibrosis, and there is intolerance of fat in gall-bladder disease. It is important not to equate these and other conditions with food allergy. Fourth, under certain conditions some foods cause metabolic problems; a good example of this is hypoglycemia (low blood sugar) brought on by the ingestion of carbohydrate foods. Once again, this is not food allergy. A fifth factor may be food additives: whether they can cause problems has been a matter of concern brought to the forefront in the last few years. And last, there is genuine food allergy.

The symptoms of food allergy can vary from occasional minor discomfort to frequent life-threatening problems. A symptom may start on the first day of life; it may remain solitary or be associated with other allergic symptoms.

The symptoms are varied, including itching and swelling of the lips, sores in the mouth, vomiting, gaseous distension, cramps, diarrhea, hives and headache. Some symptoms, such as those in the mouth, may appear instantly on contact with the offending food, whereas others may not start until an hour or so later.

There does not seem to be a one-to-one relationship between cause and effect; in other words, the offending food may produce symptoms of allergy only now and again and not every time. Certain foods produce allergic symptoms only when they are eaten in sufficiently large amounts. In some people the food causes symptoms only when a combination of events takes place; e.g., the ingestion of an offending food combined with exposure to, say, a pollen the person is allergic to or along with physical or emotional stress. Thus, a person may complain of an itchy palate while eating melon only during the ragweed season. Some foods create problems when eaten raw but not when cooked; cooking somehow alters the structure of the food and makes it less allergenic.

DIAGNOSIS OF FOOD ALLERGY

The diagnosis of food allergy is made mainly by history. In some people the relationship between the ingestion of food and the development of symptoms is so dramatic that no further information is needed. For instance, if a person gets hives each time he eats fish or a child has a swollen lip every time he eats peanut butter there is little doubt this is food allergy. Such people very often do not even consult their doctor and they probably need not. Then there are people who get recurrent symptoms such as hives or abdominal pains where food allergy is strongly suspected but not proven. And there are the people in whom food allergy is not commonly suspected or even thought of but when no other cause can be found food allergy is invoked as a possible cause.

When food allergy is suspected, a careful history is the most essential tool in making a diagnosis, and perhaps the most important part of the history is an accurate food diary. If your symptoms are sporadic or episodic, write down everything you ate in the preceding 48 or 72 hours. It is important to list not only the kinds of food but also the brand names. If symptoms are almost continuous, you must keep a daily food diary. Your doctor will examine you very carefully, for it is important to rule out other diseases that may mimic food allergy.

The value of allergy skin tests in food allergy has been overemphasized. Quite often, even with an undisputable history of food allergy, the results are negative. Therefore, although positive results are useful, negative results do not rule out food allergy. The most reliable method of tracking down food allergy is an elimination diet.

Elimination Diet

Diets of any kind can be dangerous, particularly for children, because of alterations in nutritional content. Do not undertake an elimination diet until you have discussed this with your doctor or pediatrician.

In its simplest form this diet consists of eliminating the suspected food for at least 3 weeks, and reintroducing it in usual amounts in the fourth week. If the symptom in question disappears when the person is off the food and reappears when the food is reintroduced, the diagnosis of food allergy is made.

Another type of elimination diet is one that eliminates groups of foods rather than single items. For example, you could avoid milk and dairy products, then cereals, then legumes such as peas, beans, and nuts, and so on.

A strict elimination diet is one in which the person is maintained on a basic diet of rice and pineapples, and one new food is added every 3 days or so. Obviously such a diet is used only for very troublesome conditions where food allergy is suspected, and is carried out only under strict medical supervision with nutritional assays.

Other Tests

Allergy tests are not very helpful in the diagnosis of food allergy. Both false negative and false positive results can occur. The RAST test, which is a blood test, has been tried in making the diagnosis of food allergy but with equivocal results. Finally, there is a type of test in which an extract of the suspected food is placed under the tongue and the pulse rate is measured. At present, this test seems too empirical to provide any definite clues to food allergy.

TREATMENT

The only treatment for food allergy is avoidance of the offending food or groups of foods. If the symptoms are life-threatening or serious these foods must be avoided for the rest of the patient's life. If the symptoms are less troublesome an attempt may be made to reintroduce the food every 6 months or so. Antihistamines do not relieve gastrointestinal symptoms produced by food allergy but may control hives. Sodium cromoglycate (which is used to prevent symptoms of rhinitis or asthma) has also been used to prevent symptoms of food allergy; the medication must be taken orally for this purpose. Hyposensitization therapy, which works so well for inhalant allergies and insect-sting allergy, cannot be given for food allergies.

MILK ALLERGY

One of the first allergens the potentially allergic child encounters is cows' milk. Milk has been romanticized by poets and pushed by nutritionists as the almost perfect food, and a strong lobby of dairy farmers advertises "cold beautiful milk" and "thank you milk." But there is no getting away from the fact that cows' milk is a foreign protein and a very potent allergen to the newborn child.

Whenever possible an attempt should be made to breastfeed the newborn. There is definite evidence that this reduces the chances of allergic symptoms developing in the child, and breast milk has many other advantages. Cows' milk, in any form, should be delayed until 6 to 9 months of life. If a mother cannot breastfeed her baby, formula milk is a good substitute, as it resembles human milk. But goats' milk, being the nearest to human milk, may be the best substitute.

Milk allergy is a child's first encounter with allergic diseases. The manifestation in an infant can be dermatological in the form of eczema, or gastrointestinal, or as nonspecific symptoms such as irritability and failure to thrive. The eczema can vary in severity from a few patches of dry skin to widespread redness, dryness and peeling. The commonest gastrointestinal symptoms are colic, distention, gas and vomiting, and either constipation or diarrhea; the latter may progress in some cases to a fulminating type of colitis, with bloody stools. I have seen some children who are so allergic to milk that one drop placed on their skin, or milk that they regurgitate, produces hives.

Diagnosis

Once the diagnosis of milk allergy is made, the treatment will be simple. The problem very often is that milk allergy has just not been considered as a cause of the symptoms; in other words, the diagnosis is not going to be made unless you or your doctor suspect that this is milk allergy. Milk-allergic children rarely need to see an allergist, although intradermal skin testing will yield a positive result.

The best test for milk allergy is trial and error, or better called elimination and rechallenge. Milk must be eliminated for at least 2 weeks. If, during this period of abstinence from milk, there is a dramatic improvement in symptoms, no further tests are needed. If, however, the results are doubtful, the child should again be given milk in the usual quantities; if he is allergic to milk his original symptoms should reappear.

Treatment

As soon as milk allergy has been diagnosed in a newborn infant, a milk substitute must be chosen. Soya milk is a good substitute and should be the first choice. Soya-based infant formulas are readily available from drug stores but are stocked by very few supermarkets. They tend to be slightly more expensive than regular formulas. Most newborn infants accept soya formula quite readily, some may object to its taste for a little while, and only a few will reject it altogether.

Once the infant has been started on soya milk, one of two problems will arise.

Some children thrive on soya milk initially but then experience symptoms of allergy to this too. These are similar to those due to cows' milk. Once again, the best test for suspected soya allergy is elimination and rechallenge. If the child is truly allergic to soya milk, he must be nourished on a synthetic predigested formula. These formulas usually contain predigested milk protein along with sucrose, tapioca starch, corn oil and essential vitamins and minerals. Such formulas are even more expensive than soya milk, but this is considered a prescription nutrient and may be covered by your drug insurance plan.

If a child is doing well on a milk substitute, the question is when and how to wean him from this and reintroduce cows' milk. No rules of thumb can be given. I feel that the substitute should be continued for anywhere from 6 to 12 months and at the end of this the infant should be challenged with cows' milk once again. If the child does not tolerate cows' milk, then of course he must be put back on the substitute. If, however, he does tolerate the milk, cows' milk should be gradually introduced into his diet.

ADULT TYPE OF MILK ALLERGY

The adult form of milk allergy (which, incidentally, is also seen sometimes in children), manifests itself in rather vague symptoms. Gastrointestinal symptoms may or may not be present. Instead, the patient may have respiratory symptoms, like nasal stuffiness, frequent infections, catarrh and sometimes even asthma. This form of milk allergy is not as dramatic as the infantile form, and therefore may not be suspected for quite a long while. Allergy skin tests are sometimes positive. Certain blood tests may indicate milk allergy in adults (milk precipitins). Elimination, however, is the best test.

An adult with proven milk allergy must avoid milk and all dairy products. Avoidance must be complete.

It is important to stress that some form of milk is present in many foods. Therefore, the following foods are **prohibited**:

Creamed soups, and most commercially available soups, prepared luncheon meats, cheese, pies, butter, custards, puddings, cakes, cookies, biscuits, candy, chocolate, bread, desserts, gravies and sauces.

Foods that are **allowed** are:

All fruits, all vegetables, home-made soups, clear soups, home-made bread, crusty rolls, rye bread, gelatin desserts, home-made cookies, non-dairy creamers, all meats and fish, poultry, and eggs.

If you plan to embark on a milk-free diet, you must spend time working out a balanced menu. Fortunately, in an average adult who is otherwise healthy, the absence of milk from his diet does not lead to nutritional deficiencies and therefore does not call for any other nutritional supplement.

Unfortunately, there are no guidelines to tell you how long you should be off milk. It has to be a process of trial and error. I suggest that you reintroduce milk every 3 to 4 months and make a careful note of your symptoms and reactions. Some people have to remain on this milk-free diet for the rest of their lives, whereas many others are able to go back to a relatively normal diet.

WHEAT

Next to milk, wheat is the commonest source of food allergy. At the outset, it is important to make the distinction between allergy to wheat and intolerance of wheat. The distinction sometimes is only academic, for at times the two conditions can have identical symptoms and treatment of both is essentially the same. Wheat intolerance, also called celiac disease, is caused by an inability of the body to digest a certain portion of the wheat (gluten), possibly because of an inborn error of metabolism. Allergy to wheat, however, like any other allergic process, is caused by an antigen–antibody reaction in your system, with liberation of histamine. Wheat allergy is seen in three settings.

First, the commonest situation is the infant who reacts to the first spoon of cereal with a rash, abdominal colic, or diarrhea. Here the diagnosis is obvious and hardly any diagnostic tests are needed.

Second commonest is when there is no clear-cut history of wheat allergy in infancy, but an older child or adult has troublesome eczema or asthma which is made worse by the ingestion of wheat and wheat products. The diagnosis here is not that obvious and requires a higher index of suspicion. Proof is obtained by a combination of allergy tests and elimination diet.

The third situation is where wheat acts as an inhalant that has entered the body through the respiratory system. This is seen in bakers and millers and occasionally in housewives. It causes a condition called baker's asthma. Some allergists do not accept this as a true wheat allergy, believing it to be an allergic reaction to molds on the wheat.

Wheat shares its antigenic quality with other cereals, mainly rye, barley, and oats. Therefore, a wheat-allergic person may be allergic to these other cereals also. The treatment of wheat allergy is, once again, avoidance. The avoidance must be complete, which by no means is easy, as wheat is present in one form or another in many foods and beverages — in bread, cookies, biscuits, all pasta preparations (spaghetti, etc.), malt, some prepared meats, soups, beer, cream of wheat, wheat germ, gravy and pies.

Once again, with wheat as with other food allergens, the duration of abstinence from wheat must be decided individually and by trial and error.

EGGS

Egg is a very potent allergen and can cause the whole spectrum of symptoms. It is capable of causing the most violent allergic reaction, including the dreaded anaphylactic shock. The culprit is usually egg white, and very rarely the yolk. Egg allergy usually starts early in infancy.

Egg-sensitive children may be allergic to chicken. They also have to be careful with vaccines that are grown on egg embryo, including those against influenza, mumps, measles and rabies. Avoidance of eggs has to be complete: for some patients who are supersensitive to eggs, even breaking an egg in the kitchen can engender a shock-like state. I strongly recommend that eggs not be bought at all in such households.

NUTS

Nuts are a potent source of food allergy. Just about any nut can cause allergic reactions, the commonest being peanuts, almonds, hazelnuts and walnuts. It is interesting that although the peanut belongs to the legume family, it cross-reacts with other nuts.

Because nuts can produce very severe reactions, any evidence of allergy to them should be taken seriously and all nuts and foods containing nuts (such as cookies, cakes, and margarine) should be completely avoided. Persons who have significant reactions should avoid nuts completely for the rest of their life.

SPICES

Although spices can cause true allergic reactions, it is difficult to be sure sometimes whether the reaction is allergic in origin or just an intolerance of the spice. A number of spices are capable of causing allergic reactions; mustard, pepper, and vinegar are perhaps the commonest offenders.

VEGETABLES

Once again, probably any vegetable can cause allergic reactions. Reactions are commonest with peas, beans, and tomatoes. Sometimes the allergic reaction to either peeling or cutting a vegetable is by inhalation rather than eating; the inhalant on the vegetable is very often a mold and sometimes pollens. As with milk, raw vegetables may cause greater reactions and the same vegetable in a cooked form may be more tolerable.

MEATS

Among the meats, beef, pork and chicken are the commonest culprits and lamb is the least common. Prepared meats contain not only meats but also spices, milk, and cereals.

FISH AND SHELLFISH

These are among the more potent allergens. Violent reactions occur in some allergic individuals. There is cross-reaction between the various kinds of seafood, and therefore one must be careful in eating any kind when there is a well-documented history of seafood allergy. In people who have had significant reactions to any kind of seafood, I recommend that they avoid fish and shellfish for the rest of their life.

ALCOHOL

Alcoholic beverages can cause genuine allergic reactions. However, it is worthwhile remembering that alcohol increases the flow of blood in the skin and the nose, and therefore a sense of congestion in the nose along with warmth of the skin may not represent a true allergic reaction. Most alcoholic beverages contain, besides alcohol, ingredients such as cereal, yeast, molasses, malt and spices, and therefore, an allergic reaction to an alcoholic beverage could come from any of those ingredients.

CORN

Corn allergy manifests itself in the gastrointestinal tract, the respiratory system, or the skin, depending on the mode in which it enters your body. Corn is extremely widespread and is present in the following foods and articles.

Foods: Baking flours, cakes, cookies, breads, pastries, pies, jams, jellies, puddings, soups, sauces, dressings and gravy, beer, whisky and liqueur, candy, ice cream, corn sugar, corn starch, corn oil, popcorn, carbonated beverages and prepared meats.

Articles: Envelopes and stamps, cosmetic powders, starch in clothes.

Medications: Many medications contain corn as inert vehicles.

MISCELLANEOUS

Honey, coffee, chocolate and certain gums (used in manufactured candies and ice cream) are sometimes responsible for allergic symptoms.

FOOD ADDITIVES

The whole question of allergy to food additives is surrounded by controversy and many questions are still unanswered. There are several hundred, possibly even thousands of additives we may (wittingly or unwittingly) ingest — starting with fertilizers and insecticides applied on the farm and including chemicals used to improve the appearance of fruits and vegetables, hormones and antibiotics fed to animals before slaughter, preservatives, flavoring and coloring agents, texture agents and tenderizers, and chemicals used in curing, processing, canning and packing.

The exact mechanism of untoward effects of these food additives on the body is not known. Is it a chemical or toxic reaction or is it a true allergic reaction? Does one food additive react with another in our body? And what are the 'safe' levels of these additives in our foods? Food additives have been implicated in many diseases, but exact proof is lacking except in the case of monosodium glutamate (MSG) in relation to the so-called 'Chinese-food syndrome.' Some of these diseases are the chronic tension–fatigue–anxiety syndrome, headaches, dizziness, emotional disturbances, the hyperactivity and learning-disability syndrome, chronic urticaria, and of course cancer.

The following foods usually contain additives. Read the labels!

1. Prepared meats and poultry, preserved meats and poultry, cured meats, luncheon meats, canned fish and meat.
2. Ketchup, mustard, mayonnaise, pickles, relish, salad dressings.
3. Jams and marmalades.
4. Gelatin desserts, ice cream, puddings, flavored yogurts.
5. Fruit-flavored drinks, 'ades, soft drinks; some bottled and canned 'pure' fruit juices and concentrates; instant milk drinks.
6. Candies, gum, confectionery.
7. All bakery products, including bread.
8. Instant soups; canned soups, vegetables, and fruits.

9. Colored butter, peanut butter, fats, oils, shortening and margarine.
10. Processed cheese.
11. Instant cake mixes, many commercially available flours, instant mashed potatoes.
12. Ales, wines, cider, lager, malt liquor and liqueurs.
13. Snack foods, chips, and cheese sticks.
14. Instant tea and instant coffee.
15. Many breakfast cereals.

What is there left to eat? You are probably right — not much. The following diet has a minimal additive content. Try it for 3 weeks or so, and if you experience some improvement you might want to continue it a little longer. It is worthwhile remembering that a new diet may have a 'placebo effect' (a psychological improvement due to the introduction of anything different); therefore, you must be as objective as possible.

1. Home-prepared meats and poultry products without meat tenderizers; home-made soups.
2. Fresh fruits and their juices.
3. Fresh, well-washed vegetables (even better if home-grown).
4. Home-made dressings, ketchup, and pickles.
5. Home-made bread, cookies, and desserts.
6. Cottage cheese, plain yogurt, buttermilk and milk.
7. White butter and natural peanut butter.
8. Regular tea and percolated coffee.
9. Selected breakfast cereals, oatmeal, and cream of wheat.
10. Honey; home-made jams and jellies (without addition of commercial fruit pecctin).
11. Spaghetti with home-made sauce, home-made pizza.

The following is a list of **food additives** and the foods in which they are commonly found. But remember these may change — **read labels!**

1) PRESERVATIVES

Sodium and Potassium Nitrate Smoked sausage, ham, luncheon meats; some cheeses

Sodium and Potassium Nitrite Preserved meats and poultry; side bacon

Sodium Sulphite Wines, cider, beer; canned tuna; biscuit dough, instant potatoes; dried fruit

Benzoic Acid, Sodium Benzoate Tomato paste, ketchup, pickles, relish, marmalade and jam, pickled fish

Butylated Hydroxyanisole (BHA), Butylated Hydroxytoluene (BHT) Dried breakfast cereals, dehydrated potatoes; dried beverage mixes; fats, oils; chewing gum

Sodium and Potassium Bisulphite, Sodium and Potassium Metabisulphite Ales; wines; tomato puree; dried fruit; commercial fruit pectin (for making preserves at home); "pure" reconstituted lemon juice

Propyl Gallate Margarine, fats oils, shortening; dried breakfas cereals; chewing gum

Sodium Propionate Breads cheeses; cured meats, fish, an poultry

2) SWEETENERS

Saccharin

3) FOOD COLORINGS

Amaranth Red no. 3 Bread, but ter (not margarine), cheese concentrated fruit juice, marma lade, jam, ice cream, icing sugar liqueurs, flavored milk drinks pickles, smoked fish, tomat ketchup, dried breakfast cereal and snack foods

Erythrosine Same as Amaranth above

ndigotine Same as Amaranth, above

Sunset Yellow FCF Same as Amaranth, above

Tartrazine Yellow no. 5 Same as Amaranth, above

Brilliant Blue FCF Same as Amaranth, above

Fast Green FCF Same as Amaranth, above

Citrus Red no. 2 Orange skins only

Ponceau SX Maraschino cherries, glacé fruits and fruit peel only

Caramel (natural) Same as Amaranth, above, plus pickled fish and meats

4) FLAVORINGS AND FLAVOR ENHANCERS

Vanilla, almond, lemon and artificial flavors like fruit, buttermilk, spearmint (Food labels list whether natural or artificial but are not required to specify the flavor or flavor enhancer used); Bakery products (except bread), some buttermilk, candies, chewing gum, cocoa, ice cream, instant soups, medicine, potato chips, powdered fruit drinks, pop.

Brominated Vegetable Oil Citrus or flavored drinks

Caffeine Cola drinks

Tannic Acid Cider, wine, honey wine; chewing gum

Monosodium Glutamate (MSG) Canned soups, canned vegetables, fish, meat. Sold as a spice, it may be added in any amount in restaurant meals and prepared and ready-cooked foods.

Salicylates Ice-cream, bakery goods (except bread), candy, chewing gum, soft drinks, gelatin desserts, jams, cake mixes, wintergreen-flavored products

5) TEXTURE AGENTS

Propylene Glycol Salt

Alum Pickles, relishes, baking powder, flour, starch, liquor, ale and lager

Epichlorohydrin Starch

Carboxymethyl Cellulose Salad dressing, flavored milk drinks, processed cheese, ice cream

Polyoxyethylene Stearate Bakery products

Saponin Beverage mixes, pop

Sodium Alginate Coarse salt; infants' formulas; frozen fish; ale, lager, malt liquor, flavored milk drinks, cream, cheese, ice cream, mustard

Acacia Gum (Gum Arabic), Tragacanth Gum Ice cream; processed cheese, skimmed milk, mustard pickles

6) DOUGH BLEACHING, MATURING, AND CONDITIONING AGENTS

Benzoyl Peroxide Flour

7) GLAZES AND POLISHES

Mineral Oil Confectionery

Shellac Candies, cake decorations

8) EXTRACTION AND CARRIER SOLVENTS

1,3-Butylene Glycol Flavors

9) ENZYMES AND YEAST FOODS

Calcium Carbonate (chalk) Bread

10) MISCELLANEOUS

Polyvinylpyrrolidone Ale, lager, cider, wine

Paraffin Wax Fresh fruits and vegetables (especially thick coating on root vegetables sold out of season); cheese

HYPERACTIVITY, LEARNING DISABILITY, AND FOOD ALLERGY

A few years ago Dr. Benjamin Finegold shook the world with his hypothesis that hyperactivity and many learning disabilities were caused by a reaction to food additives and natural salicylates in food. Over the years Dr. Finegold's theory has been both hailed and refuted by responsible researchers. At first there was some disbelief and scepticism about this theory, but gradually nutritionists, pediatricians, psychologists and allergists realized that this hypothesis was not altogether wrong. The whole syndrome of hyperactivity and learning disabilities is complex and it is probably too simplistic to account for it on the basis of food additives alone. I feel that, if hyperactivity or an unexplained learning disability is significant, a diet containing neither food additives nor natural salicylates (*see* Aspirin Allergy for list of foods containing natural salicylates) might be tried for at least 3 months. If it seems to help, perhaps it could be continued a while longer. If it doesn't, it should be discontinued. In any event, seek the advice of your doctor or pediatrician. Diets can be dangerous, particularly for children, because of changes in their nutritional content.

There is no doubt the diet is complicated. Any mother who has been advised to try her child on this will do well to study the diet first and make a shopping list of the necessary ingredients. She will probably find more of these ingredients in health-food stores and food co-operatives than in supermarkets. (Prices are usually lowest at co-operatives.)

It is usually a good plan to start the entire household on this diet initially: not only does this overcome the potential problem that the child will feel 'different' but also it makes life a lot easier for the mother! It is important to make careful observations while the child is on this diet and try it for at least 3 months before coming to any conclusions.

This is my modification of the Kaiser–Permanante diet. The following are **prohibited.**

(1) FOODS

Fruits: apple, apricot, all berries, cherry, grape, currant, raisin, nectarine, orange, peach, plum, prune.

Vegetables: tomato and cucumber

Nuts: almond

Cereals: all cereals with artificial color and flavoring

All instant breakfast preparations

Baked goods: all ready-made cakes, cookies, rolls, pie crust, and frozen baked goods

Many bake mixes

Meats: all prepared meats such as bologna, salami, frankfurters, sausages, and so on

Poultry: prepared turkey, commercially cooked chicken

Seafood: frozen fish and shellfish that has been dyed or flavored

Ready-cooked meals: TV dinners and 'fast foods'

Desserts: all commercially produced ice cream, pudding, sherbet, custard, flavored yogurt, dessert mixes

Candies: all commercially produced candies

Beverages: all colored soft drinks, all diet drinks, commercially available milk shakes, tea, commercially available chocolate milk, frozen and instant orange juice; all instant drinks; cider, wine, beer, punch, coffee

Herbs and Spices: prepared mustard, commercial vinegar, salad dressings, sauces, cloves, ketchup

All colored cheese

Polyunsaturated margarine and colored butter

(2) NON-FOOD
Items not allowed
All toothpastes and tooth powder, mouth washes, lozenges (use bicarbonate of soda as a mouth-cleanser) and cough drops
All vitamin preparations
Any medication containing acetylsalicylic acid (ASA)
Perfumes

The following foods are allowed. For home-made items, use ingredients from this list
All vegetables except tomato and cucumber
Fruits: Banana, pineapple, grapefruit, pear and lime, fresh, or home-made into juices, jellies, and jams (without commercial fruit pectin)
All cereals without artificial color or flavoring
Home-made cakes and cookies (without artificial coloring)
Meats prepared at home without additives; home-made soups
All poultry not commercially prepared.
Eggs
All fresh fish and shellfish
All desserts made at home without artificial coloring or flavoring
Home-made custards and puddings
Home-made candies (without almonds)
Home-made lemonade; non-colored and non-flavored soft drinks
Milk, plain yogurt, buttermilk
White cheese and white butter, cottage cheese
Home-made mustard and mayonnaise, distilled white vinegar

All commercial breads (except whole-wheat and egg bread)
All flours
All cooking oils
Home-made chocolate syrup; pure maple syrup
Honey

12

URTICARIA

HIVES! HIVES!

Hives (urticaria) remains one of the most perplexing problems for the allergist. More often than not it turns out to be nonallergenic in origin.

Urticaria is characterized by small, rounded, raised swellings of the skin, accompanied by redness and itching. Sometimes, however, the swellings may be large, either from the start or when many small swellings have merged to create big ones; this is called giant urticaria. Urticaria may be accompanied by swelling of certain parts of the body, such as the lips, tongue, hands and feet; this condition is termed angio-edema. A very rare but sometimes severe and potentially dangerous symptom of urticaria is laryngeal edema, in which the vocal cords become swollen and the patient has great difficulty breathing. The underlying mechanism of all forms of urticaria is the same; namely, the release of histamine in the skin and subcutaneous tissues.

Histamine can be released in the body tissues by large numbers of specific and nonspecific stimuli, and the stimulus is not necessarily allergic in origin. This is why it is so difficult to determine the exact cause of hives in many cases. (In 75% or more of cases of recurrent urticaria, the exact cause remains unknown.) In children, however, urticaria usually is allergic in origin and very often the allergen can be traced. Some of the causes of urticaria are:

1. *Physical causes*, such as cold, heat (produced by activity or by exposure to sunlight), and water (this is rare). Certain drugs, such as tetracycline, diuretics, tranquilizers and sulfa medications, predispose patients to photosensitivity.

2. *Emotional causes*, such as panic, anxiety, or depression, can lead to troublesome urticaria.

3. *Food*. Hives can be due to allergy to any food but is commonest after the ingestion of hyperallergenic foods, such as nuts and seeds, eggs and chicken, fish (especially shellfish), peas and beans, and citrus fruits. Also, food additives can be a cause of urticaria.

4. *Drugs*. Any drug allergy can cause hives, but the common drugs responsible for this are ASA (Aspirin, etc.) and other pain remedies, laxatives, antibiotics and tranquilizers.

5. *Systemic disease*, either overt or covert, can be accompanied by hives. In particular, hives develops in patients who have one of the collagen group of diseases or intestinal parasites.

6. *Dermatographia*. This condition is characterized by hives; it develops in response to stimulus-like pressure

on the skin. Common causes of pressure on the skin that may cause hives include tight-fitting clothing, carrying a heavy bag, contact with a powerful jet of water, rubbing the body with a towel, scratching, and handling vibratory tools.

7. *Other allergic diseases.* Hives sometimes occurs in association with other allergic diseases such as rhinitis or asthma.
8. *Insect bites and stings* can lead to local or generalized hives.
9. There is an extremely rare urticarial-like condition that is hereditary. This is caused by an inherited deficiency of a certain blood protein. The lesions are not red and during attacks the gastrointestinal system is affected.

The cornerstone in the diagnosis of urticaria is a careful history. Physical examination and blood tests will eliminate any underlying diseases. Allergy tests are of very limited value — even when food allergy is suspected, a food diary and elimination diet are more useful than allergy tests. In maintaining a food diary, write down everything you ate during the 4 to 6 hours preceding the onset of hives. Make sure to check labels of frozen and canned foods, and include food additives in your diary. The doctor who advises you to try this diet will probably eliminate groups of foods rather than single foods for 3 weeks at a time.

Chronic or recurrent urticaria of unknown origin is by far the commonest type of hives and can affect as high as 20% of the population. It helps to look on this condition as a state of altered body chemistry rather than an allergy. The human body is a living laboratory of chemicals, minerals, enzymes and hormones, all of which function in harmony in the normal state. Even a slight imbalance in these chemicals may lead to hives. The condition by itself is not serious, but it is frustrating for both the patient and the doctor and searching for the elusive cause only increases the frustration. Very often it is a self-limiting condition and seems to disappear as mysteriously as it started.

The following measures should help in alleviating chronic or recurrent urticaria.

1. Discuss the condition with your family doctor. His examination and tests should reveal or eliminate any underlying disease.

2. Avoid or reduce excessive physical and mental stress. Try to get an extra hour of sleep and reduce some of your weekend activities.

3. Reduce irritation of the skin by avoiding sources of pressure such as tight-fitting clothing or footwear.

4. Avoid ASA and other pain pills, laxatives, tranquilizers and other over-the-counter medications. (See Chapter 15 for information about medications that contain ASA.)

5. Avoid histamine-releasing foods such as strawberries and bananas. Also avoid foods that contain natural salicylates (See Chapter 15). It may be worth trying a 3-week elimination diet that avoids food additives.

6. Take an antihistamine regularly. If the hives have a set periodicity, it is a good plan taking the antihistamines ahead of time. If the hives are unpredictable, try to take the antihistamine every 8 to 12 hours. If the antihistamine makes you drowsy, take it at least nightly.

13

DRUG ALLERGY

CAUTION! I'M ALLERGIC TO THAT

During the last decade there has been an overwhelming increase not only in the number of medications available but also in our use of these medications. And this applies not only to prescription drugs but also to over-the-counter medications. There is no doubt that we are a drug-oriented society. And along with this increase in drugs has come an increase in adverse reactions to the drugs. In addition there has been a vast increase in the types and number of chemical substances used in medical investigation. Statistics can vary, but some authorities claim that as high as a third of all diseases are caused by drugs.

There are various types of reactions to drugs and it is important to realize that not all of them are allergic in origin.

First, there are side effects, which every drug can produce if given in sufficient doses; for example, if you experience drowsiness with antihistamines, this is a side effect. Second, there are idiosyncrasies, whereby a particular drug produces an unpredictable effect. For example, some patients — particularly children — become hyperactive and excitable after taking antihistamines, and some people vomit or have a headache after taking certain analgesics. These are examples of idiosyncrasies and not true allergic reactions. Third, there are toxic effects; these usually relate to strong medications such as anticancer drugs. And last, of course, there are true allergic reactions.

A true allergic reaction to a drug is manifested by a rash, which can be either a red measly rash or hives. In very severe cases the skin may peel.

If you are intolerant of certain drugs it is important you sort out this intolerance with the help of your doctor. To do this you need to know the exact name of the medication or, failing this, the prescription number and the name of the pharmacy where the drug was purchased. In addition, you must describe clearly the symptoms that developed and their time sequence. When you have all this information it is imperative that you establish two points with your doctor. First, was the reaction a true allergic reaction? And second, if in the future you may need to take this drug, can you or can't you take it?

Many patients loosely call a drug reaction a drug allergy. This label is carried by word of mouth for several years, and eventually the exact details of the event are forgotten. In such cases, the patient may be unnecessarily depriving himself of a medication that he may need and is not allergic to.

The diagnosis of drug allergy is made principally on the basis of a good history. Allergy skin tests, similar to those done for hay fever, are of some help. Other more complicated and expensive laboratory tests are becoming available, and in the years to come may be widely used and more meaningful.

Allergy can develop to just about any drug but is more commonly seen with the following: antibiotics, analgesics, sedatives and tranquilizers, laxatives, hormones such as insulin, diuretics and other antidiabetic drugs, certain medications used in special x-ray procedures, horse serum and some vaccines.

There is no definite relationship between being an allergic person and having an allergy to drugs. However, I recommend all allergic persons to be very careful with any medications they take and to make careful notes not only of the medication they are on but also of any reactions they experience.

Some authorities recommend patients with known drug allergies to wear a bracelet or similar identifying object, and many patients seem to derive a sense of security from this. This is discussed under Allergy and Bracelets in Chapter 16.

ALLERGY TO SERUM

There are two types of allergic reaction to serum. The immediate (anaphylactic-type) reaction consists of a rash and difficulty breathing; this can develop within minutes and may be serious. A delayed version of allergy to serum is called serum sickness and develops in a matter of days or weeks and consists of joint pains and fever. The delayed version is rarely life-threatening.

The commonest serum in use today is horse serum for the prevention of tetanus (antitetanus serum). It is usually administered after trauma. If you are allergic to horses or have a history of genuine allergy to horse serum, you should never be given this type of antitetanus serum and should receive human antitetanus serum instead. Also, you *must* maintain your antitetanus immunity by regular administration of tetanus toxoid.

ALLERGY TO VACCINE

It is important to point out that a local reaction such as redness, swelling, pain and even fever after the administration of a vaccine is not an allergic reaction but a toxic one. A reaction to a vaccine should be considered an allergic reaction only if it is accompanied by a generalized rash or wheezing.

All live viral vaccines are grown on chick or duck embryo; therefore, patients who are allergic to eggs are most likely to be allergic to these vaccines. They include the vaccines to protect against measles, mumps, rubella, influenza and rabies. The best test for egg allergy is whether you can eat an egg safely: if you have no problems with this you are not allergic to eggs and can receive these live viral vaccines.

PENICILLIN ALLERGY

Allergy to the various forms of penicillins is perhaps the commonest type of drug allergy. About two decades ago this was the most dreaded allergy to drugs; accounts of fatal reactions were common. Today, penicillin allergy is common in all the developed countries but it is seen in a different form; the commonest manifestation is a rash. It is important to point out that nausea, vomiting, and diarrhea while you are taking penicillin do not constitute allergy to this drug — these are side effects.

The diagnosis of penicillin allergy is made chiefly on a good history. Therefore, it is important that you record carefully any symptoms that develop while you are taking this drug. Taking a Polaroid picture of the rash is an even better idea, for not all rashes brought on by penicillin are allergic in origin. In particular, rash is a common symptom due to a type of penicillin called ampicillin, but this is thought to be nonallergic in origin.

Very many people have been labeled as allergic to penicillin either because they have been told this and never to take penicillin again or they have come to this conclusion (probably erroneously) on their own. For the vast majority of the generally healthy population it doesn't really matter, because probably they will never need to take penicillin. However, some people have a frequent need for antibiotics — for example, those who have allergic respiratory problems, cystic fibrosis, or other chronic systemic diseases where frequent infection is a problem. For these people it is important to be sure whether they are allergic to penicillin.

You should take time to recollect and record all the facts surrounding your true or alleged allergy to penicillin and discuss it with your doctor. Allergy skin tests to penicillin are of limited value: a negative result does not altogether rule out the possibility of penicillin allergy, but a positive test will help. If you are in fact allergic to penicillin and need antibiotic therapy frequently for infections, or you are unfortunately subject to a life-threatening disease for which penicillin is necessary, you can be desensitized to the drug. This desensitization to penicillin can be done only in a hospital.

ASPIRIN (ASA) ALLERGY

Acetylsalicylic acid (ASA, a trade name of which is Aspirin) is perhaps the commonest drug responsible for allergy. Nausea and heartburn are side effects of ASA and should not be considered an allergic manifestation. A genuine allergy to aspirin manifests itself by rash and swelling of areas of the body. ASA allergy develops in association with nasal polyps and bronchial asthma in some people, and this drug also seems to cross-react with some non-ASA analgesics and anti-inflammatory drugs. Patients allergic to ASA may also be intolerant of certain foods containing natural salicylates, and of certain food additives (e.g., sodium benzoate and tartrazine yellow dye no. 5).

The following foods contain natural salicylates: apricots, berries, cherries, currants, grapes, nectarines, peaches, plums, prunes, tomatoes and cucumbers. The following foods contain salicylates as flavoring agents: ice-cream, bakery goods (except bread), candy, chewing gum, soft drinks, gelatin desserts, jams, cake mixes and wintergreen-flavored products.

ASA is contained in many types of medications; for example, analgesics, headache pills, backache pills, and remedies for stomach upsets, menstruation problems, sinusitis, colds, and so on. The following is a list of medications containing ASA: Alka Seltzer, Anacin, Ascriptin, Aspergum, Bromo-Quinine, Bromo-Seltzer, Bufferin, C1, C2, C3 and C4 tablets, Coricidin, Darvon compounds, Disprin, Dristan tablets, Empirin, Excedrin, Fiorinal, 4-Way Cold tablets, Midol, Norgesic, Novahistex with APC, Novahistine with APC, Pepto-Bismol, Phenaphen compounds, Robaxisal, Talwin compounds, Veganin, and the compound tablets numbered 217, 222, 282, 283, 292, 293, 294 and 692.

Acetaminophen (Tylenol, Tempra, Atasol) can be used as a substitute for ASA in the majority of cases. Do not exceed the recommended dose.

ALLERGY TO LOCAL ANESTHETICS

Local anesthetics such as those used in dentistry can cause problems such as fainting, palpitations, and some swelling at the site of the injection. These, however, should not be regarded as allergy to the anesthetic substance — true allergy to the drugs is extremely uncommon. If you suffer from any of these symptoms during or after dental work, I suggest you go well rested for your dental treatment and perhaps take a tranquilizer beforehand. Also, it is important to rest in the dentist's office for about half an hour or so after the treatment.

14

ENVIRONMENTAL CONTROL

MAKE YOUR HOME A HAVEN

The cornerstone of treatment of any allergic condition is the avoidance of offending allergens or reduction in exposure to them. The avoidance of foods, insects, and contact allergens is discussed in the appropriate sections. In cases of respiratory allergic conditions, like rhinitis, sinusitis, and asthma, control of the immediate environment is an important consideration — and environmental control measures must begin at home. Some patients go to the extreme, expending large sums of money to create an allergen-free home. This is not necessary; but with a proper understanding and some effort it is possible to make your home a haven.

HOUSE DUST

House dust is the commonest antigen — it is always present. The first step in treatment should be its reduction and control.

"Isn't everybody allergic to dust?" and: "There's not much I can do about dust at home, is there?" are the questions I am asked most frequently when I counsel patients about the control of house dust. No, not everybody is allergic to dust (although most of us are intolerant of it); and yes, there is a lot you can do to reduce dust in your home. It is important to realize, however, that not all dusts are allergenic although most dusts are irritants.

House dust is not just the dust you see on a tabletop. It is what your vacuum-cleaner bag contains; namely, a combination of dirt, upholstery, rugs, drapes, human and animal hair and skin, feathers, mold, household insects, cement and plaster, and so on.

The Patient's Bedroom

A good place to start dust-control measures is the bedroom. Keep the room generally bare and free of clutter and have only the basic furniture. Chenille creates lint and is best avoided. Hang washable curtains or plastic blinds at the windows. Rugs are best avoided; if one is needed, use a washable cotton mat or a removable synthetic carpet. Do not have books, pictures, or toys in the bedroom; allow only one washable stuffed toy on the bed. Feathers should be strictly avoided; pillows, cushions, quilts and eiderdowns are common sources. Store clothing outside the room or in garment bags in closets. If the patient has the windows closed while he is sleeping, ventilation can be provided through an exhaust fan in the window (blowing outward) or, preferably, an air-conditioner.

Bedding is a storehouse of dust. A relatively new mattress is preferable, with a zip-on cover (which will contain the dust) or a thin plastic sheet covering it. Cotton thermal blankets are preferable to wool or synthetic blankets; they are not only warm but also easily washable.

The bedroom floor and furniture should be vacuum-cleaned thoroughly daily — and don't forget to vacuum under the bed and inside the closets. Clean with a moist cloth; do not apply wax — this only attracts more dust. Once a week, take the bedding apart and beat and vacuum-clean the mattress. Clean the hot-air registers thoroughly by dropping the flexible hose of the vacuum-cleaner into the duct as far as it can go, then cover the registers with cheesecloth or an old nylon stocking.

Basement Rooms

The basement is another source of dust. Activity in an unfinished basement should be restricted, as this can be particularly dusty. The floor and walls should be painted if possible. Woodwork and weaving are sources of allergenic dust and are best avoided.

Hot-air furnaces should be cleaned frequently. Washable filters are preferable to disposable ones; they should be washed or cleaned at least once a week. During the colder months, proper humidification is extremely important: it is important to maintain the humidity in your home between 40 and 45%. If you have a hot-air furnace, a proper central humidifier is recommended — most humidifiers that come with furnaces are inadequate. Alternatively, you must maintain one or more portable cold-mist humidifiers in your home. Electronic air-cleaners, despite popular belief and their manufacturers' claims, do *not* reduce dust significantly. (They do remove some circulating dust particles from the air, but how can they remove dust from your rugs, drapes, and mattresses?) Your best plan is to get a good vacuum-cleaner, keep it accessible, and use it often.

AIRBORNE POLLUTANTS

A person allergic to dust is highly intolerant of airborne pollutants such as smoke, sprays, fumes and smells, and every attempt should be made to reduce these in the home. This is covered in the Air Pollution section.

DANDER

Complete avoidance of all fur-bearing animals and feathered pets is absolutely essential if you are allergic to dander.

Perhaps this is all that needs to be said about dander allergy, but man's love for animals usually precludes a rational understanding of the mechanism of this condition. To provide an understanding of dander allergy it would not be out of place to restate some basic principles of allergic reactions.

1. There is always a latent period between the first exposure to the allergen and the development of symptoms. This answers the frequently asked question: "I have had my dog for 2 years, so why am I allergic to it now?" Another common question is answered by this same principle of the latent period; it is: "We got the dog for a trial period of 2 weeks and nothing happened during that time." The exact latent period cannot be specified and may vary from a few days to years.

2. Exposure to two or more antigens can compound the allergic effect. For example, if you are allergic to dust and pollen, the introduction of a dog or cat may make your original symptoms worse. This explains the statement: "I had my symptoms even before I got my dog."

3. Exposure to the offending allergen may not invariably provoke the symptoms. To put it another way, on some days the dog can sit on your knee and you will not notice any symptoms but other days even going into the same room as the dog may make you sneeze or cough.

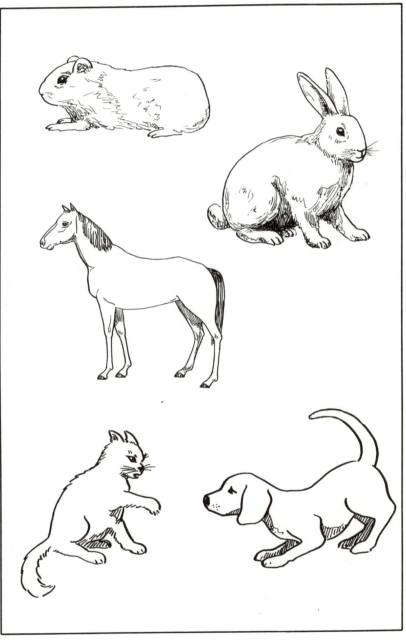

4. With perennial antigens a certain amount of tolerance or reduction in the severity of acute symptoms may develop, but this should not be understood as indicating immunity or absence of allergy to that allergen. The offending allergen, even though it does not cause dramatic symptoms, produces a low-grade but constant inflammation of the respiratory tract, making you susceptible to nonallergic respiratory symptoms and respiratory infections. Therefore, parents whose child does not evidence any clear-cut symptoms while they have a pet should understand that allergy to the animal may manifest itself as recurrent upper respiratory tract infections or unexplained wheezing. The belief held by some patients that they are not allergic to their own dog but only to another dog is fallacious.

5. The severity of symptoms of any allergic condition can depend upon the amount of exposure to the allergen. Symptoms of animal-dander allergy are experienced most often in the middle of the night, and more in the winter (when the central heating is on and the animal is more confined to home).

6. The allergen responsible for dander allergy can be hair (or feathers), skin, or saliva, or a combination of all three. Poodles, even when devoid of fur, have skin and therefore are not nonallergenic. It is difficult to compare the allergenicity of different animals; therefore, it is difficult to say whether a boxer is more allergenic than a terrier, or whether a pedigree Siamese cat is more allergenic than a stray tabby.

7. Central heating creates air currents; hot air rises, and cooler air takes its place. These air currents can carry dander from one part of your home to another, so it makes little sense to confine your pet to the basement and hope that you have solved the problem.

These statements make it clear that, if your allergy tests indicate you are allergic to dander, and if you understand the basic principles of dander allergy, you will be well advised not only to get rid of your pets but also to avoid any further exposure to them outside your home. Barns, farms, stables, circuses, zoos, and sleigh-rides must be avoided. Visits to homes where there are dogs or cats will have to be avoided, even at the risk of upsetting your social life; in the warmer months, a child who has dander allergy may be able to visit his friend or play outside the friend's home, but in the colder months he must have the friend visit him instead.

Dander can be very adhesive. It can stick to clothes, drapes, linen, upholstery and rugs; these items should be washed thoroughly, or cleaned (if possible, professionally), after the pet has gone. Remember that dander can be brought into the home on clothes and luggage, and from so-called outdoor pets. Also, many outdoor pets come in to eat or spend the night.

I realize that getting rid of pets is not easy. There will be frustration and unhappiness in letting them go, but your health will benefit immeasurably. (Giving the pets to a friend or relative whom you know will care for them can make the experience a little less traumatic for the family.)

ALLERGY AND FUR

Contrary to popular belief, fur coats do not cause allergy even to people who are allergic to animal dander. This is because the fur is not living hair and does not produce dander. However, a fur coat can cause irritation around the neck, and the dyes and other chemicals used in processing the pelt can cause dermatitis.

NEWSPRINT

Some patients have quite distressing symptoms on exposure to printed matter — books, magazines, newspapers, computer printouts, etc. With newspapers, the problem may be solved by changing to a different one. Patients who are intolerant of all newspapers may have to wear a mask while reading them or place the printed paper underneath a transparent plastic sheet.

POLLENS

The common pollens responsible for allergic symptoms are those of grasses, trees, and weeds. The times of pollination depend upon geographic location and variations in seasons from year to year. Generally, trees pollinate in spring, grasses in late spring and early summer, and weeds in late summer and early autumn. Pollens are present at all times of the day and night but usually are in heaviest concentration in the air very early in the morning and late at night. During the pollen season, therefore, outdoor activities after supper should be restricted. Rain prevents pollens becoming airborne and washes them away.

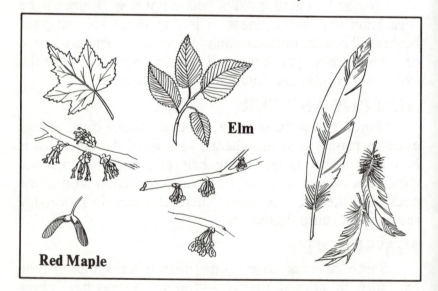

It is very difficult to eliminate pollens completely from one's environment, but having the windows closed when you are sleeping does reduce the pollen count in your bedroom.

Sufferers from pollen allergy should exercise some caution in selecting a place for summer vacations (see Holidays, in Chapter 16). Likewise, someone with pollen allergy is well advised not to undertake an outdoor summer job.

MOLDS

Molds or mildew are a common cause of respiratory allergy. They are present throughout the year but certain kinds predominate in the spring and fall, when the snow is about to thaw and when it is about to come.

Molds can develop wherever there is moisture. There are many types, a common one being the growth of green and white spots on bread, etc., left in a closed container. Molds on foods such as cheese do not cause respiratory symptoms.

Allergenic molds are found mostly in the soil. Molds thrive on decaying vegetation, and therefore grow in great abundance in places such as farms, barns, and stables — and piles of leaves in your garden. Thus, activities that increase your exposure to molds include raking leaves, living in damp accommodation (e.g., summer cottages), playing in old caves, and hiking through damp wooded areas.

Inside your home, molds are likely to develop in a damp basement. This can be discouraged by cleaning the basement floor and ensuring that it is always dry. The waterpan of a humidifier is another source of mold and therefore should be kept clean at all times. If there are moldy spots in your home, treat them with a solution of equal parts of bleach and water.

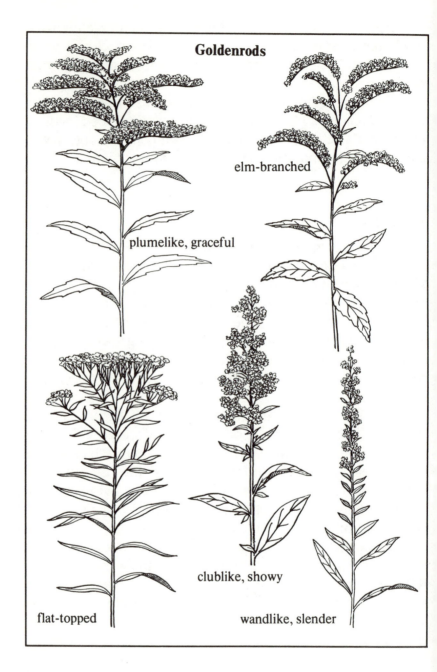

Goldenrods

elm-branched

plumelike, graceful

clublike, showy

flat-topped

wandlike, slender

Houseplants harbor molds, so are best avoided or reduced; the pots of such plants should be kept clean and the soil covered with sand or pebbles. Cut flowers may carry outdoor molds and should be avoided. At Christmas time an artificial tree is preferable.

AIR POLLUTION

The word 'pollution' is heard very often but, for the allergic patient, it has a rather specific meaning. He is concerned mainly with airborne pollution, the type that affects his respiratory system from the top of his nose down into his lungs. Modern civilization has added a lot of pollutants to the air we breathe; these are harmful to most people but particularly troublesome to allergic persons. However, it is important not to consider as allergic those symptoms that are caused by the inhalation of pollutants (irritants).

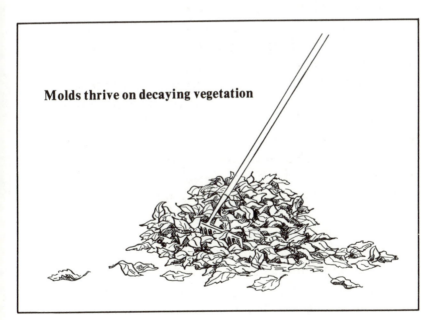

Molds thrive on decaying vegetation

Intolerance of pollutants is not allergic in origin, although the allergic person suffers more than the non-allergic. It is therefore proper to say: "I am intolerant of perfumes," rather than to say: "I am allergic to perfumes." One cannot receive allergy injections for pollutants, and anti-histamines and decongestants may not help very much. However, treating the underlying allergic condition will gradually decrease intolerance of pollutants.

The list of pollutants that can trouble an allergic person is endless. It includes such obvious things as tobacco smoke, automobile exhaust, and fumes from industrial plants, but also such common household items as aerosols, paints, polishes, waxes, varnish, cleansers and detergents, glue, cooking odors, disinfectants and deodorizers, insect repellents and insecticides, perfumes and cosmetics, and the smell of newspapers, books, newly dry-cleaned garments, and any other substance with a strong odor. Symptoms on exposure to these pollutants can vary from patient to patient. In some it may cause redness and tearing of the eyes; in others, nasal stuffiness and discharge and sneezing; and in some others it may bring on an attack of asthma.

It is practically impossible to have a home free from pollutants, but every effort should be made to reduce them. Smoking in the allergic patient's home (and car) should be strictly prohibited. Avoid aerosols — use pump sprays whenever possible, and roll-on deodorants rather than the aerosol type. Avoid the unnecessary use of chemicals. It is better to paint your home in the summer, when the windows can be kept open; if at all possible, the allergic patient should stay out of the home while painting is in progress and for at least a couple of days afterward. By the same token, an allergic patient should not visit a newly painted home. A fireplace with an improperly functioning chimney can add a lot of smoke to your home: have it checked. A central electronic air-filter does help to reduce household odors; portable electronic filters are almost useless.

Outside your own home you can do only so much, but the allergic person should avoid bonfires, campfires, and polluted places as much as possible. For example, department stores, supermarkets, and restaurants are sources of pollutants for the allergic. Thus a person might find himself sneezing when walking by the soap and detergent aisles, or in clothing shops — fabrics and clothes emit a lot of strong smells because of the chemicals they contain. Restaurants abound in cooking odors and tobacco smoke.

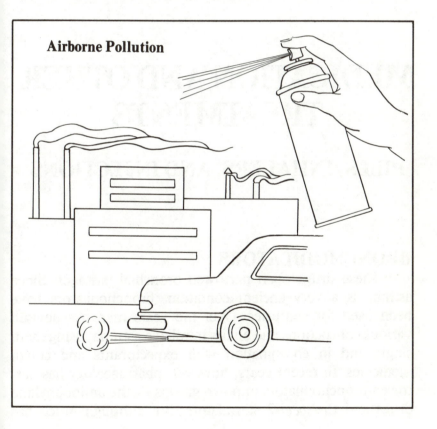

Airborne Pollution

15

MEDICATION AND OTHER TREATMENTS

PILLS, INHALERS, AND INJECTIONS

BRONCHODILATORS
These drugs open narrowed bronchial passages. Since asthma is a very ancient condition, bronchodilators have been used for centuries. Over the years man has devised various concoctions and elixirs to relieve asthma, using them singly and in combination with expectorants and cough medicines. In recent years, however, pharmacology has narrowed bronchodilators into two groups — the aminophylline drugs and the *beta*-2 stimulators. But although much has

been learned about the mechanisms of these drugs in asthma, the exact action is still unknown.

The aminophylline drugs are available as pills, liquids, suppositories, and solutions for intravenous administration. The *beta*-2 stimulators are available as pills and liquids and as inhalant mist (in nebulizers).

Despite claims by drug manufacturers, almost all bronchodilators do have some side effects. First, they may cause stomach upsets, which can take the form of nausea and vomiting or heartburn. Second, they all stimulate the central nervous system to some extent, an effect that may manifest itself as tremors, irritability, insomnia and (especially in children) hyperactivity. Third, they all share the ability to induce palpitations. However, most of the side effects can be avoided if the drugs are used judiciously.

There are two basic ways in which bronchodilators can be used.

1. The asthmatic whose symptoms are sporadic should take bronchodilators only when a bout of asthma is anticipated or present.
2. The patient whose asthma is present all the time or recurs frequently should take bronchodilators every 4 to 6 hours throughout the day. (A general rule of thumb is that if you wheeze more than twice a week you should take bronchodilators regularly.)

The choice of bronchodilator depends upon individual variation in patients and also their physicians. Some patients can relieve their wheezing quite successfully with one type of bronchodilator, whereas others may do better on a combination of both the aminophylline and the *beta*-2 stimulator types.

Remember: bronchodilators taken orally start working in about 30 minutes and the effects last 4 to 8 hours, and you must not stop taking the drug immediately the wheezing becomes inaudible (because the smaller air passages within the lungs may still be obstructed). My general advice is that bronchodilators must be continued for at least 48 hours after all wheezing has stopped.

Patients who wheeze only sporadically and can predict its onset should take bronchodilators before the episode starts. Thus, a child who wheezes each time he has a respiratory infection should start taking his bronchodilator as soon as infection develops, even if there is no wheezing. Likewise, the person who wheezes on exposure to cold air, or during or after exertion, will do well to take his bronchodilator ahead of time.

Aerosol Inhalers (Nebulizers)

Beta-2 stimulators are available in various forms, including aerosol mist in a nebulizer. Over the past decade these asthma inhalers have become very popular, but their use requires an understanding of their limitations and dangers and also the proper technique for using them.

The dangers from these asthma inhalers stem from two factors:
1. Because their action is almost instantaneous it is very easy to misuse them. It is not uncommon for a person with severe chronic asthma who has been using an inhaler several times an hour to be rushed in death-like condition to a hospital emergency department.
2. These hand-held asthma inhalers are powered by a propellant, the effects of which on your system are still not completely known.

Therefore, oral preparations of bronchodilators (pills or liquid) should be used for long-term therapy and asthma inhalers should be reserved for emergencies. Also, you should never use a nebulizer more than 3 or 4 times a day. If you find yourself using it more often, consult your doctor immediately.

It is very important that the inhalant be used with the correct technique. Otherwise, the medication is lost in the air and does not enter the lungs. I recommend the following procedure.

1. Shake the inhaler. Remove the protective mouth-cap. Insert the mouthpiece in your lips and purse your lips tightly around it.
2. Take 1 or 2 breaths with the inhaler in your mouth.
3. Exhale completely. Inhale deeply; as you start this, press the nozzle-button of the inhaler. As you complete the inhalation, take your finger off the button.
4. Remove the inhaler from your mouth. Keep your lips closed, and hold your breath as long as possible.

An alternative way to use these hand-held inhalers is as follows.

1. Hold the inhaler just outside your mouth and *do not* purse your lips around it — keep your mouth open.
2. Breathe out.
3. Breathe in, and at this instant press the nozzle-button of the inhaler.
4. When the puff of medication has gone into your mouth, close your mouth and hold your breath as long as possible.

The inhaler's plastic mouthpiece must be washed at least once a week. *Do not* insert a pin or needle into the jet inside the mouthpiece.

Initially you may have a problem determining whether your inhaler is empty. The inhaler delivers 200 metered aerosols; therefore, the best bet is to keep a count of how many puffs you have had. The mist may decrease in size or force with use, and the bottle within the inhaler will gradually feel lighter.

In hospital, bronchodilators may be administered by a process called wet nebulization. The medication is in liquid

123

form and is given through a mask attached to a small gadget. The advantage of this is that the medication reaches the smallest part of your respiratory tree and, being in droplet form, works much better. Some patients who wheeze a great deal and need to visit a hospital frequently for such treatments may be recommended to rent or purchase a respirator of this type and use it at home.

CROMOLYN SODIUM (Sodium cromoglycate)

It is not very often that one sees a drug which arrives with a lot of fanfare and not only lives up to its reputation but does even more, a medication that is a definite milestone in therapy. One such drug is cromolyn sodium (also called sodium cromoglycate). It comes in three forms; namely, Intal for inhalation into the lungs, Rynacrom for insufflation (puffing) into the nose, and Opticrom as eyedrops.

Like many one-of-a-kind drugs, cromolyn sodium has an interesting history. Many years ago, while in Egypt, a British researcher came upon a group of natives smoking a cigarette made of the leaves from a certain plant. His curiosity was aroused, particularly when he discovered that many of the smokers were asthmatic and that their symptoms improved after they started smoking. It did not take long for the scientist to realize that there was a potentially useful drug in this leaf, but it took several years of painstaking research to identify the chemical agent, synthesize it, and make the drug commercially available.

Cromolyn sodium is a true preventive drug and its action is unique. It is not an antihistamine, nor a cortisone, nor a bronchodilator. When inhaled or insufflated, it coats the cells of the membrane that lines the respiratory tract. This prevents the release of histamines from these cells after an allergic reaction has taken place. The active substance stays on the lining of these cells for 4 to 6 hours and then disintegrates. It therefore follows that cromolyn sodium will be most efficacious if it is:

a) taken ahead of time; and

b) repeated 3 or 4 times a day, as long as the allergic person is exposed to the allergenic substance.

No side effects of cromolyn sodium have been reported so far. The only problems I have seen with the drug are as follows.

1. Cromolyn has to be taken with a gadget (a Spinhaler for the lungs, and an insufflator for the nose), and very young children may have difficulty using this. However, I have seen children as young as 3½ or 4 years managing this with some help and encouragement from their parents.

2. There may be some mild tickling of the nose or throat as the drug first enters your system. This is very short-lived and does not pose a serious problem. (a) In the case of Intal, you can relieve the tickling by drinking some water. (b) With Rynacrom, the sensation can be overcome by sniffing — do not blow your nose. (Sniffing spreads the medication into the back of the nose; blowing your nose would expel the medication.)

3. Cromolyn sodium is expensive. You should be aware of the cost of this treatment at the outset.

Cromolyn sodium prevents symptoms that are brought about by allergic reactions. Therefore, it works best when one is dealing with a purely allergic condition. If allergy is absent or not very prominent, or the condition is a mixture of allergy and infection, the drug may not be very efficacious.

Cromolyn Sodium for Your Lungs (Intal)

From the foregoing description you will realize that this drug is effective in the treatment of pure allergic asthma, less so for mixed asthmatic conditions, and perhaps not at all for intrinsic or infective asthma. Thus you will also realize that Intal works best in younger asthmatics, as opposed to asthma developing later in life; by the same token, Intal provides most relief in cases of well-defined allergies such as to pollens, molds, or dander.

To be effective, Intal must be started before the onset of the allergic season. For example, if you are allergic to grasses, you must start taking Intal about a week or so before the grasses start pollinating, use it throughout the grass-pollen season, and continue for a week or two after the end of the season. Asthmatics who are allergic to most pollens and molds should take their Intal from the time snow disappears in the spring until the first frost in the fall. When you discontinue Intal, don't do so abruptly; taper off the treatment gradually.

Before you start using Intal, you should know how a Spinhaler works. It has two parts: the main body with a gray sleeve, and a mouthpiece along with the propeller. The medication is in the form of a capsule. Insert the capsule, with its colored end downward, into the propeller. Screw the body of the Spinhaler into the mouthpiece and then move the gray sleeve down once and up once. (Without this movement, the Spinhaler will not deliver the medication into your lungs.) Next, hold the Spinhaler in your fingers like a cigarette, and breathe out to empty as much air as possible from the lungs. Tilt your head back, place the mouthpiece between your teeth and purse your lips around it, and breathe in deeply through the Spinhaler as quickly as possible. Hold your breath for a few seconds, then breathe out through the nose. You may have to repeat this procedure once or twice. Then remove the Spinhaler from your mouth, open it, and check that the capsule is empty. (A few particles of medication may remain in the capsule, but this is not important.)

Wash the parts of the Spinhaler at least once a week. It is recommended that a Spinhaler be replaced after about 6 months of use. Keep the medication in a dry place: the powder cannot enter your lungs if it gets caked in the capsule.

Intal can be used in conjunction with any other medication for your asthma, such as bronchodilators. It is basically a preventive medication and does not abort an acute attack of asthma. If anything, if you take Intal during an acute episode of wheezing, your wheezing might get worse. If you are wheezing badly, it is preferable to take a bronchodilator and wait about 30 minutes or so before using Intal.

Some asthmatics respond so well to Intal that they require no other medication, whereas others need additional medication such as bronchodilators. You must use Intal for at least a month before you decide whether it is doing you any good. If, after a month, you feel that neither the severity nor the frequency of the asthmatic episodes has decreased, probably Intal is not suitable for you.

Cromolyn Sodium for Your Nose (Rynacrom)

The same basic principles apply to Rynacrom as to Intal. Rynacrom is very effectual in cases of seasonal allergic rhinitis (hay fever), less so in perennial allergic rhinitis, and perhaps not at all in mixed allergic and vasomotor rhinitis.

It is best to start using Rynacrom just before the onset of your allergic season, and continue using it throughout the season and for a few weeks afterward. If you have hay fever symptoms throughout the spring and summer, you should take Rynacrom from the time the snow disappears until the first frost.

Originally, Rynacrom was available as a powder to be used with an insufflator. Very recently it has become available as a nasal solution in a squeeze bottle. Insert 1 or 2 drops of the solution in each nostril about 4 to 6 times a day. For milder types of hay fever, twice a day is sufficient.

Rynacrom can be used safely in conjunction with other medications for rhinitis, such as decongestants and antihistamines. It may soon be available as a nasal solution, which would make it a lot easier to use.

ANTIHISTAMINES

'Antihistamine,' as the word suggests, works by destroying the histamine that is released from your cells in response to an allergic reaction. Theoretically, antihistamines should work for all types of allergic reactions and provide virtually complete relief from symptoms. In fact, this was the expectation when this type of medication first became available. However, over the years we have found that antihistamines work in only very limited circumstances. Exactly why this happens is not known, but one possible reason is that antihistamines cannot destroy the other chemical substances that an allergic reaction releases along with histamine.

The antihistamines are most helpful in upper respiratory allergic conditions but less so in lower respiratory ones. Thus they relieve the symptoms of rhinitis and sinusitis but are not very effective against the symptoms of bronchitis and asthma. These drugs also alleviate the itch of allergic eczema and provide short-term relief in the case of hives. Antihistamines are a part of almost all cough medications. They help reduce an allergic type of cough but are of no use against a nonallergic cough.

Antihistamines are made up in various forms — pills, timed-release capsules, syrups, creams and injections. They are generally safe but do have some side effects.

Side Effects

The biggest drawback to antihistamines is the drowsiness they cause, an effect that is quite variable but is invariably greatest when you start using them. Some people can take as many as 6 antihistamine pills a day and experience little if any drowsiness, whereas others become extremely drowsy after taking only half of one. When you start on these drugs it is wise to take them only at bedtime and then increase the dose gradually. More important, until your body has adjusted to the medication — and permanently, if you experience any drowsiness at all — while taking antihistamines you should not drive or engage in activities that demand vigilance and attention. Also, do not drink alcohol if you take antihistamines.

Another problem with antihistamines is the development of tolerance. This means that a particular antihistamine will relieve your symptoms for a while but then will gradually lose its effectiveness. If this happens, you can try two remedies: (a) increase the dose (for example, instead of 2 or 3 pills a day, take 4 to 6 a day); and (b) change to another brand of antihistamine.

Although antihistamines normally have a sedative effect, some or all brands have the opposite effect in certain individuals: a child may become hyperactive and an adult may not be able to sleep. Again, a change of brand may solve the problem.

The effects of antihistamines taken during the first 3 months of pregnancy are not known for certain. Therefore, it is prudent not to take them at all in early pregnancy and to avoid them as much as possible throughout.

Antihistamines can potentiate the effects of alcohol. This is why people who are taking antihistamines should not drink alcohol.

Apart from these side effects, antihistamines are perfectly safe even in children. They are not habit-forming and, if they seem to help, there is no reason why you cannot take them for any length of time.

Which Antihistamine Is Best?

Most antihistamines can be bought without a prescription. Many of my patients ask which antihistamine I recommend, but I can only tell them the best is the one that works best for them. It is really a question of trial and error before you find one that is best suited to you.

CORTISONE

Cortisone, the wonder drug of the century, does wonders for allergies too. However, it is a hormone and a very potent drug and should not be used lightly: it should be reserved for acute and life-threatening emergencies or for very disabling and severe symptoms. Therefore, the drug is almost never used for upper respiratory conditions such as hay fever or allergic rhinitis. In bronchial asthma, when everything else has failed we resort to the use of cortisone; but here again, every attempt should be made to take as little of the medication as possible. If your doctor advises long-term use of the drug, he will probably recommend an alternate-day schedule.

A cortisone preparation (Beclomethasone) for use in an inhaler is now available. Although it has less side effects, one should use the inhaler with the same respect and caution accorded other forms of cortisone. Your doctor will probably recommend that you reduce the dose of cortisone gradually when you are going off the drug.

Some of the side effects from the prolonged use of cortisone are a gain in weight, swelling of the feet, peptic ulcer, diabetes and softening of the bones.

One should never use cortisone lightly or without a proper schedule. Popping a pill of cortisone now and again is gross misuse of this drug.

Cortisone cream is particularly useful for eczema and contact dermatitis. Again, it is important to choose the right kind of cortisone in the right kind of ointment base. If the eczema or dermatitis is severe, a good way to ensure that the cortisone stays on the skin is to wrap the area in a piece of plastic overnight.

Cortisone Inhaler for the Lungs

In resistant, intractable cases of asthma, when all other medications have failed and long-term cortisone therapy is needed (which will have side effects), use of a cortisone inhaler for the lungs should be considered. If nothing else, this treatment should enable you to reduce the number of cortisone pills you have to take. You must use the inhaler regularly 3 or 4 times a day, and it will be at least 2 weeks before you notice any appreciable benefit.

Even in the inhaled form, cortisone is absorbed into your system (through the lining of the respiratory tree) and therefore should not be used indiscriminately. Inhalations of cortisone may produce a fungus infection in the throat, causing some discomfort and soreness. If this happens, the inhaler must be discontinued and cortisone pills substituted until after the infection has cleared. Also, during periods of stress or infection you may have to supplement the inhalations with cortisone pills.

Nasal Cortisone Inhaler

Like other forms of the drug, nasal cortisone sprays must be used intelligently and properly. Obviously, these sprays are not suitable for every nasal condition. The prime indication for their use is chronic intractable perennial allergic rhinitis, with or without sinusitis. The words 'chronic' and 'intractable' are important: you do not use a cortisone spray for a condition that is of only short duration, and every other form of treatment must be tried first. There are 3 or 4 types of cortisone nasal sprays; all are equally efficacious.

Cortisone nasal sprays do not provide instantaneous relief — they must be used for at least a couple of months before you can see any change. Also, one must not use them excessively, as they are absorbed through the nasal mucous membranes and, over a period of time, cortisone can build up in your system.

There are many treatment schedules. I prefer my patients to take 2 puffs twice a day in each nostril for 2 months, then none for 1 month, and repeat this schedule for at least 6 months. If this seems to be helping them, I suggest they continue this regime for at least a year.

Cortisone nasal sprays should not be used by pregnant women or infants, and by older children only under medical or close parental supervision.

Apart from a short-lived nasal irritation, cortisone sprays have no side effects if taken as directed.

ALLERGY INJECTIONS

Allergy injections (desensitization or hyposensitization therapy) were begun as an empirical method (i.e., based on experience) for the treatment of allergic conditions. Over the years the technique has been refined and today we know a lot more about it than we did even 2 decades ago. To put it simply, allergy injections produce a different kind of antibody in your system, called the blocking antibody, which interferes with the antigen–antibody reaction that develops in response to an allergen.

These injections are effective against only 2 types of allergic condition, inhalant allergy and stinging-insect allergy. Of the conditions caused by inhalant allergens, hay fever probably responds the best; perennial rhinitis comes next, then asthma in which the allergic component is significant. Bronchial asthma caused mainly by infection will not respond to allergy injections. Also, hyposensitization does not relieve conditions such as allergic eczema, which may be associated with conditions such as rhinitis and asthma. There are injections that reduce allergy to stinging insects but not biting insects, and none for food allergy or contact dermatitis.

Only a doctor, or a registered nurse under a doctor's direct supervision, is allowed to administer allergy injections. Nurses are not allowed to give them on their own outside a doctor's office. The injections are given in the lower part of the upper arm, and it is advisable to have all the injections in the same arm. Before you receive each allergy injection, it is advisable that *you* identify *your* vial. It is important that you remain in the doctor's office for 20 minutes after the injection; before you leave, have your arm checked by the nurse and make sure of your next appointment. For about 2 hours after the injection you must not engage in any sport or activity that gets you overheated, as this would speed up absorption of the allergy serum and might cause a reaction.

Allergy injections can be very beneficial. If they are taken for the right reason, and with the right attitude, and of course with the correct technique, they are bound to help.

The Allergy Serum

The allergy serum is usually sent to your doctor, or to the clinic where the injections will be given. Sometimes, however, it is mailed to the patient. If this happens, as soon as you receive the serum you should check the bottles to see whether they are cracked. If a vial is cracked, return the entire box of vials at once. If the vials have frozen in the mail, stand the package in the fresh-food section of the refrigerator and let them thaw. Allergy serum must be refrigerated at all times. (Leaving it at room temperature shortens its lifespan). Because the serum is a suspension of many different ingredients, it may contain small particles and/or not be completely clear. However, there should be no large particles and the serum should not be very cloudy; the only exceptions to this rule are certain aluminum-precipitated vaccines, which are milky. Most allergy serums are valid for about 1 year; the expiry date is indicated on the vials.

Unlike most medications, allergy serum is handmade individually for each patient; therefore, no 2 serums are identical. The serum is made up in a set of 3 or 4 or 5 vials, which contain the same solution but in different dilutions: vial 0 or 1 is the most dilute, and vial 3, 4 or 5 the most concentrated.

The best time to begin allergy injections for seasonal allergies is in the fall. Starting injections for hay fever in the spring will not help you that year, as it takes about 4 to 6 months before allergy injections start producing their beneficial effects.

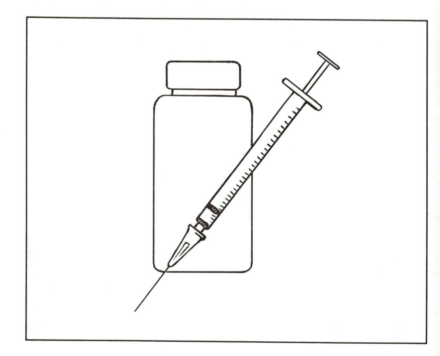

Treatment Schedule

Treatment usually begins with a small dose given weekly, starting with the most dilute serum and working upward until the maintenance dose is reached. Then, a booster injection is needed every 2 or 3 weeks. You must have the injections for at least 2 years, and your response to the treatment should be re-evaluated by your doctor at least every 2 to 3 years.

It is very important that you attend regularly for your allergy injections: irregularity not only reduces the efficacy of the injections but also makes you more likely to have a reaction. Therefore, whenever your injection schedule has been interrupted you must point this out to the nurse administering the next injection, as the dosage has to be appropriately reduced.

• Do not take your allergy serum with you on a short trip or holiday.

• If your injection schedule is interrupted for more than 3 months you must start it all over again.

• A slight cold should not prevent you getting your regular allergy injection. But you should skip a week if your temperature rises above 100°F (37.5°C) or you have a cough and wheeze.

• If you move but will be living in the same general area, you can take your allergy serum with you; keep it as cool as possible during the journey. Find another doctor, and continue injections with as little interruption as possible.

• If you move to a different area, it is best to discontinue the injections for a while. Find a doctor in the new area, and have yourself retested after you have been in that environment for a few months.

• If you change over from serum made by one laboratory to that made by another, you have to start at the smallest dose and work up the doses all over again.

135

- The injections can be continued during an otherwise normal and uncomplicated pregnancy, as there is no evidence that these injections have any harmful effects on the unborn child. But you must consult your obstetrician about this. If there are any complications during your pregnancy, however, or you have a history of difficult pregnancies, it is advisable to discontinue the injections.
- If you are to continue with a second or subsequent series of injections, make sure your allergy serum is reordered in good time. Be aware that, even if you continue on the same serum, you have to restart on a weekly schedule: the newly made-up serum, being fresh, may be stronger than the old serum.

Reactions to Allergy Injections

Some amount of redness, itching and swelling at the site of the injection is common. When we talk of swelling after an allergy injection we mean the raised, hive-like swelling, surrounding the site of the injection. This local reaction is usually short-lived. (I prefer that my patients have a local reaction, as this helps me to monitor the treatment much better.) If the local reaction is troublesome, applying an ice pack to the arm will help. Also, taking an antihistamine earlier in the day of the injection reduces the reaction. If the local reaction exceeds the size of a silver dollar, or if it persists more than 48 hours, you must bring this to the attention of the nurse or doctor.

Another type of reaction after allergy injections is what is called the focal reaction. This causes symptoms such as nasal blocking and congestion on the day of the injection and for about 24 to 48 hours afterward. Such focal reactions are common when you start the course of injections but they tend to disappear on their own. If they are troublesome, take an antihistamine earlier in the day of the injection and perhaps the next day.

The most serious reaction to an allergy injection is what is called the systemic or anaphylactic reaction. This consists of a generalized rash or urticaria, along with wheezing, choking, some stomach pains, plus a feeling of 'passing out' and diarrhea. *This is a medical emergency and must be treated as such.*

INJECTIONS FOR ALLERGY TO INSECT STINGS

Patients who experience troublesome or serious reactions to insect stings should consider desensitization to these insects. (There is no therapy for desensitization to insect bites, such as mosquito bites.)

Until recently, whole-body extracts have been used to desensitize patients to insect allergy. But now, pure insect venom has become available and many allergists expect that treatment for all insect-sting allergies will be with the venom rather than with whole-body extracts. At present, however, insect venom is expensive and testing with it is cumbersome.

INSECT-STING FIRST-AID KITS

Anyone who is significantly allergic to stinging insects should carry a suitable first-aid kit or have easy access to one. The essential items are a tourniquet, an antihistamine tablet, and a syringe containing a solution of epinephrine. You can buy the kit complete or make it up yourself. The medications in the kit should be changed every year and replaced immediately if used.

REPOSITORY ALLERGY INJECTIONS

Repository injections are absorbed extremely slowly into your system and therefore need to be taken infrequently. This obviously makes repository allergy injections very attractive, but it is important to point out that (at least in my experience) they are less efficacious and likely to create more reactions.

The introduction of Pollinex-R, a repository allergy injection against ragweed, caused a lot of expectation and raised unrealistic hopes in some of my patients. At least in their present form, these injections are not substitutes for regular allergy injections; but for patients who are exclusively allergic to ragweed (and not to other pollens or to molds), and those who cannot take the regular allergy injections, Pollinex-R is worth a try.

Repository allergy injections for grasses, also, have been introduced recently, but I have some reservations about using these until more is known about them. Unlike ragweed, which is a single antigen, there are numerous antigenic grasses; this is one of my concerns about a repository grass-pollen vaccine.

EPINEPHRINE

An epinephrine injection is given in two acute situations. First, it is a drug of choice in an acute allergic reaction such as that produced by an insect bite or drug allergy. Second, it is also very useful in acute asthma episodes.

The drug has many actions, but basically it reduces congestion and stops an allergic process in the body. Generally, administration of this drug should be left to your doctor; but, in a dire emergency, self-administration of epinephrine may be permissible. Most people suffer palpitations, sweating, and some shaking of the hands after receiving this drug, but these effects are short-lived. People who have known heart disease should be very careful with epinephrine.

16

RAISING AN ALLERGIC FAMILY

PUT A SMILE ON THEIR FACES

A condition such as allergy, which mostly affects children and young adults and may produce recurrent and troublesome symptoms, is bound to touch upon many aspects of family life. With understanding and a proper attitude, it is possible to raise a healthy, harmonious, and happy family. But, without the right attitude, it is common to have disruptions, disharmony, and even tension in the family of the allergic.

When I compare the harmonious and the disharmonious family, the one single factor that seems to separate them is their attitude. The right attitude can come only from a proper understanding of the disease on the one hand and an abundance of patience, tolerance, concern and love on the other. It is not enough just to know what it is the person is allergic to and avoid or reduce exposure to the offending allergen; it is more important to anticipate and prepare for the problems and, even more important, to preserve the self-image of the allergic person. Even after you have acquired all the information and knowledge, the one certainty about allergic symptoms is their unpredictability. How often have I seen a family get ready for a big trip and the night before the child starts coughing and wheezing and ends up in the hospital. Or the mother has a big day at the office, and just on that day the teacher telephones her that the child has been coughing a lot and wants her to take him home. Events like this are common, and the wise parent who has an allergic child will make no plans without a contingency plan also.

From the moment of conception, a child's genes govern whether he will be allergy-prone or allergy-proof. Thus, heredity is the single most important deciding factor. If both parents are allergic, the chances that their offspring will be allergic are close to 100 per cent. The exact genetic transmission of allergic diseases is not known and therefore cannot be accurately predicted. Allergy is known to skip generations; and of course there are what are called spontaneous mutations, which cause the birth of an allergic child in a non-allergic family.

There is also some anecdotal evidence that what the pregnant mother eats, inhales, or takes by way of medication can affect the unborn child and be a factor in deciding whether that child will be allergic. I have heard some allergists say that pregnant women should not drink any milk or take any medications, including any over-the-counter preparations such as laxatives. Maybe this seems rather an extreme situation for the average expectant mother, but where there is a strong family history of allergy on both sides of the family it may be wise to heed this advice. Certainly, a child has a better chance of normal health if his mother did not drink alcohol, smoke, or take any drugs during her pregnancy.

In late infancy the child enters the age group where he might experience respiratory allergies. These are uncommon under the age of 1 year; they usually become evident in the second or third year of life, or even much later. The following symptoms should alert parents to the possibility of a respiratory allergy in their child. I think of such children as 'pre-allergic children.'

1. Recurrent and long-lasting colds, sore throats, or earaches.
2. Persistent clear or yellow nasal discharge.
3. Persistent sniffing, snoring, or nasal itching.
4. Mouth-breathing; speech and teething problems.
5. Wheezing associated with respiratory tract infections.
6. Recurrent episodes of croup.

It must be emphasized that these symptoms by themselves may not necessarily represent an allergy but may be the harbingers of an underlying allergic state. All you need to do at this stage is to keep an accurate diary of the child's symptoms, relating it not only to changes in weather and seasons but also to places and foods. Having done this, discuss the matter with your family physician or pediatrician. It is prudent to wait at least 6 months to a year before the child is taken to an allergist for allergy testing.

It is worth emphasizing, even at the cost of being accused of repeating myself, that although some children who have all of the 6 symptoms listed above may have an underlying allergy, the vast majority do not. Many parents who come to my office with a child who has had recurrent colds, convinced the child must be allergic to something, feel disappointed when told (after careful investigation) that there is no underlying allergy. The reason why only some of

141

the children who get recurrent infections are allergic is not clear. What renders a child immune to infection but another prone to them, also, is unclear. In the absence of any scientific knowledge about this immunity it is best to put it down to constitutional or individual variation. (Why is it that some children have difficulty with even simple mathematics, for instance, and others seem to be child prodigies? By the same token, some children seem to have recurrent infections and others do not.)

If you have a pre-allergic child it is wise to eliminate some potential allergens from his environment. Dust, feather pillows, flannelette sheets and wool blankets are best avoided. If you don't already have a pet, I strongly advise you not to get one. However, a family that has an allergic or pre-allergic child must steer clear of either extreme, of excessive concern on the one hand and negligence on the other. Excessive and undue concern about a child's actual or suspected allergies could make you or your child a neurotic individual.

What about the mother who works outside the home and whose child has troublesome recurrent symptoms? It may be difficult for a single parent to be available when needed by the child. It is obvious that a mother who has a demanding outside job with inflexible hours will not be able to provide the care, security, and attention that such a child needs. There will be times when the child may need to be driven to school. There will be days when a parent may have to go to school at lunchtime to give the child his medication. There will be nights of broken sleep and there will be frequent trips to doctors' offices and the pharmacy, and probably to the hospital. The working mother who is alone, or the couple who both work outside the home, will need a surrogate parent (a neighbor or grandparent, for example) to meet these demands. Obviously, a mother who does not work outside the home is available to meet these extra demands and care for her child.

Have you ever wondered why nights are so troublesome for the allergic child? First, when a person is lying down, mucus tends to accumulate in the air passages. Second, the tiny hair-like processes (cilia) in the air passages that are responsible for moving the mucus tend to be sluggish at night. Third, the level of cortisone in your body drops at night, making you more vulnerable to attacks of cough and wheezing.

HOME

Maintaining your home as free as possible of dust and allergens will be one of your first (and continuing) responsibilities. Details of this are in Chapter 14, but its importance cannot be overemphasized. Admittedly, you will be vacuuming and cleaning more than the average parent, but after the initial clean-up it should not be too difficult to maintain. Obviously, you would not want young children to do the heavy cleaning, and the allergic person must not be exposed to a lot of dust when cleaning is being done. However, older children should be expected at least to keep their own room in order.

SCHOOL

If your child has troublesome allergic symptoms, it is important that you meet the class teacher, gym teacher, school nurse and the principal and acquaint them with the child's problems and limitations. Responsibility for the administration of medication required during school hours is on you, not the school. The medications could be put in the child's lunchbox. If your child has a particularly bad day but not bad enough to keep him at home, it is a good idea to visit the school during lunchtime to check him and give him his medications. Alternatively, you could send a note to the teacher asking that your child be kept in during recess and lunchtime.

Most asthmatic children have some limitation of exercise tolerance, which may present problems with physical activities at school, such as gym; also, the gymnasium may be dusty, which will increase the problems. Unless a child's asthma is very severe, it is rarely necessary to take him out of gym altogether. The child should be encouraged to compete with himself and not with others, to take a brief rest when he needs to get his 'second wind,' and when appropriate to take medication just before or after the activity. Many asthmatic children are unable to take part in sports and other activities not because of any physical limitation but because of anxiety and insecurity.

Schoolwork may suffer for several reasons. Being up at night with cough and wheeze is bound to be reflected in the next day's work. Antihistamines and cough medications may make the child sleepy, and bronchodilators may make him anxious and shaky. An asthmatic child may have serous otitis, a condition that causes a hearing loss (see Chapter 5), and this would obviously create difficulties.

It is not easy to enforce environmental control measures in the school. Some of my patients' parents have been able to get their child's class involved in 'Project Dust Control,' but such approaches usually meet with a lot of resistance. If chalk dust bothers your child, ask the teacher to seat him as far from the blackboard as possible. School trips to barns, farms, stables, zoos and so on may have to be avoided.

RECREATION

It has been said that the family which plays together stays together. With some forethought and planning this aphorism can be applied to the family with an allergic child. There are some children who are little daredevils, who do too many activities; they may swim in the morning, play hockey in the afternoon, and skate in the evening, a regime that is bound to get them into difficulty. Others may make themselves into social recluses, refraining from participation in any activities. Obviously, either extreme is bad.

A certain amount of sports and recreational activities is advisable. Obviously, a child's own preferences as to the type of activity must be taken into account. Many of us who work with asthmatic children have found that swimming is particularly suitable for them; the only exception is the asthmatic child who has sinusitis, in whom swimming only worsens the condition. Ice-hockey, however, in our experience is particularly troublesome for all asthmatic children. An allergic child may need to take medication before activity or take his inhaler with him to the pool or rink.

HOLIDAYS

Use discretion when selecting where the family will go on vacation. Unfortunately, the school summer holiday coincides with the peak allergy season. Avoid visits to zoos, farms, barns and stables. Ragweed is endemic in eastern Canada and along the eastern seaboard of the U.S.A., but is much less in some maritime areas, on the west coast, along seashores and at high altitudes.

Do not take allergy serum with you on short trips or holidays: it should be in a refrigerator, not in the glove compartment of your car. Also, different doctors may not be very familiar with the patient's condition or his serum. However, you must take with you all the usual medications. If the allergic child is prone to infections, ask your doctor for a prescription for antibiotics in case these are needed. It is a good idea to take a nonallergenic pillow and blanket with you.

MOVING

If you are moving away from the area and you have an allergic person in your family, and particularly if he is on allergy injections, it is important to find a doctor in your new location ahead of time. If you carry the allergy serum with you, it must be kept in an icebox. Ask your doctor to give you a letter describing the symptoms and treatment, or have him forward the patient's file to the new doctor.

Whether you should continue your present allergy injections in your new surroundings depends largely on what you are allergic to and where you are moving from. If you are moving from one end of the country to the other, your present allergy serum probably won't be suitable for the kind of allergens you are going to be exposed to. On the other hand, if the move is only a couple of hundred miles, to a similar sort of area, you may be able to stay on the same serum.

A move is a good time to give up a family pet if this has been advised. When selecting your new home, consider dust and environmental control: measures that may have been impossible in your present home may be possible in the new one.

Very often I am asked by patients if a move to another town will help their allergies. There is no general or easy answer to this question, but by and large I believe that moving from one town to another will not solve your problems significantly. There are many reasons for this. First, some allergens are universal. Second, although you may have felt well while vacationing in your new town there is no guarantee that you will be symptom-free there always. Third, a move that is made merely to escape from your allergy symptoms does not eliminate your allergy-proneness; you should be coping with your allergies wherever you are. Fourth, a move may introduce new anxieties and insecurities. Finally, no town is allergy-free, even if it has acquired such a reputation; in any event, it is bound to have pollution, which is equally harmful to the allergic person.

CHRISTMAS

If a member of the family is allergic to pollens and mold, it is advisable to get an artificial tree rather than a real one. If you are visiting a family, make sure they have no pets and do take a nonallergenic pillow and blanket with you. If visitors are coming to your home, ask them not to bring their pets. Do not give pets as gifts — a well-meaning gift may be the source of many problems later on. People tend to eat more nuts than usual at Christmastime, which may create problems for those who have food allergies. In the excitement of the festive occasion, children may get hives: this is not necessarily an allergic manifestation.

SELF-IMAGE

The self-image of an allergic child may suffer in various ways. With having to take medication frequently, dropping out of gym and other activities, paying frequent visits to doctors' offices and perhaps emergency trips to hospital, an allergic child may get the feeling he is different from others and perhaps inferior to them. There are many ways to counter this. Above all, accentuate the positive: remind the child of the things he can do rather than those he can't. Explain to him that allergy is a self-limiting disease and that most children grow out of their symptoms in a few years. Show him or talk to him about other children with handicaps (such as muscular dystrophy and cystic fibrosis) who are much worse off.

Then there is the real or imagined guilt an allergic child feels in being a burden to his family and a 'wet blanket' in all their activities. This can be overcome by the family's display of love and warmth and by realistic, flexible planning of activities to include the child.

BEHAVIOR PROBLEMS

Are there any behavior problems special to the allergic child? Does the allergic child have a different personality from the nonallergic child? Does the allergic state create any specific emotional problems?

147

The answers to those three often-asked questions is "No." Any chronic disease — e.g., arthritis, seizures, cystic fibrosis — gives rise to emotional problems such as anxiety, frustration, depression, loss of self-image and so on. But if the primary condition is properly treated and accepted, the secondary emotional problems will not need any special treatment. It is rare for an allergic child to need formal psychotherapy for emotional problems.

COUNSELING PARENTS

Some parents seem defeated by the experience of raising an allergic child and are reluctant to have another baby. If you want to have another, I do not think the chances that the child will have allergy problems should discourage you. If both parents and at least one of their children are allergic, there is a strong possibility that further children will have allergies.

Some allergists believe that breast-feeding a baby and not giving him cows' milk or solid foods for the first 6 months may reduce the likelihood of allergies. When you start introducing foods to the 6-month-old, give only one at a time. Highly allergenic foods such as eggs, nuts, seeds, fish and shellfish should be introduced as late as possible.

IMMUNIZATIONS AND VACCINATIONS

Unless your child is allergic to eggs, all the usual childhood immunizations can proceed normally. If your child is allergic to eggs — the best test for this is whether he can eat an egg without breaking out into a rash or experiencing gastrointestinal symptoms — he must not be injected with live viral vaccines (which are grown on chick embryos). These vaccines include MMR (mumps, measles, and rubella), rabies, and influenza. If the initial reaction to egg is fairly strong and violent, like choking, wheezing, and a generalized rash, the person may have to avoid viral vaccines all his life. If the reaction to egg initially was not so strong, perhaps an attempt should be made to try the child on egg-white once a year or so; if he loses the reaction to egg, he can receive viral vaccines.

Persons who are allergic to horses must not be given tetanus antitoxin made from horse serum. However, allergy to horse serum does not prevent them from receiving the primary tetanus vaccination with the toxoid in the form of DPT (diphtheria, pertussis, and tetanus). More importantly, such children should maintain their immunity by boosters of the tetanus toxoid every 3 to 5 years. In the event of minor injury their immunity can be increased by a booster injection of tetanus toxoid, but if they suffer major trauma they will need human tetanus antitoxin. A human antirabies serum is now available for persons who cannot take the regular rabies vaccine.

Any serum can cause serum sickness, even if the person has no allergies.

ALLERGY AND BRACELETS

Many people get a sense of security from wearing a bracelet or necklet that identifies their allergies. This is a futile exercise in the case of allergies to substances such as pollens and molds, dust and feathers, but such a bracelet may be justified to identify life-threatening insect or food allergies or severe drug allergy.

There is a fear in the minds of many people that in the event of an accident they might be given a drug they are allergic to. However, even in an emergency, doctors and nurses make every effort to find out whether you are allergic to any medications. A list of medications you are allergic to, in your purse or wallet and in the glove compartment of your car, will not go unnoticed.

IS IT ALLERGY OR IS IT INFECTION?

In allergic disease of the respiratory system, whether rhinitis, pharyngitis, bronchitis or asthma, the dividing line between allergy and infection is rather thin. In other words, it is difficult to be absolutely sure whether a given episode of, say, a runny nose is being caused by allergy or infection. The following indicate a greater likelihood of infection.

a) Raised temperature and other constitutional symptoms, like aches and pains.

b) Change in the color of the nasal secretion, from clear to cloudy or frankly yellow or green.

c) History of exposure to an infection at home or work.

NERVOUS TICS

It is quite common for children to have mild neurotic tendencies such as sniffing or throat-clearing. If they have respiratory allergies also, nervous tics may be accentuated. These children must be handled with a lot of understanding. The tics can be very disturbing not only to the child but to the entire family, and statements such as "Stop making that awful noise" can only make things worse for the child. I don't think a psychologist or psychiatrist is needed, unless there are other, deep-seated, psychological problems. Most of these children outgrow the tics.

THE ALLERGIC CHILD'S FUTURE

Many parents wonder and worry about the future of their allergic children. Will their allergies retard their development — physical, mental, or emotional — in any way? Will allergies leave any permanent effects on their system? The answer is most certainly not: allergies do not cause permanent damage or have any adverse effects.

Most (if not all) children outgrow their allergy symptoms, even though they have the allergic state all their lives. In other words, they outgrow their early symptoms but may experience others later. This is discussed in more detail under The Natural History of Allergic Conditions, in Chapter 1.

17

YOUR DOCTOR AND HIS ALLERGY TOOLS

SPEAK THE ALLERGIST'S LINGO

SHOULD I CONSULT AN ALLERGIST?

One of the decisions when you are faced with suspected or definite allergies is whether to seek the opinion of an allergist. Your first contact must be with your family physician or a pediatrician, many of whom have a special interest or training in allergy and can help you. An allergist (a pediatrician or internist who has had special training in allergy) will be able to help you if you have the following problems.

A. *Respiratory problems*
  1. Seasonal or perennial nasal symptoms such as congestion, blockage, sneezing or running.
  2. Chronic or recurrent sinusitis.
  3. Troublesome postnasal drip with symptoms such as sore throat, throat-clearing, or hoarseness.
  4. Recurrent prolonged infections of the upper respiratory tract.
  5. Recurrent cough or wheezing.
  6. Itchy, red, watery eyes.
  7. Recurrent earache, or hearing loss.

B. *Skin problems*
  Not all skin problems are allergic in origin. An allergist can help you in regard to the following.
  1. Hives (urticaria).
  2. Atopic eczema, a condition characterized by dryness and itching in certain specific parts of the body; occurs in infants and children.
  3. Contact dermatitis (irritation of the skin on contact with allergens such as metals, rubber, etc.).

C. *Insect allergy.*
  In particular, troublesome symptoms after being stung by insects such as bees, wasps, yellow-jackets and hornets.

D. *Food allergy.*

E. *Hyperactivity and learning problems in children.*

F. *Certain vague symptoms such as fatigue, tension, and headache.*

G. *Drug reactions* (to determine whether they are allergic in origin).

VISITS TO AN ALLERGIST
You don't visit an allergist just for allergy tests, but for

an allergy evaluation. Therefore, go prepared with all the facts — and don't leave your car by a 15-minute parking meter! Your first visit will take the best part of an hour.

Preferably, wear a short-sleeved shirt or sleeveless top; this will make it easier for the nurse to perform allergy tests. For at least 48 hours before the tests, do not take antihistamines, tranquilizers, or ephedrine (which is included in some old-fashioned asthma medications): these medications suppress one's response to allergy skin tests. (Most newer asthma medications and cortisone do not interfere with allergy tests and therefore don't have to be discontinued.)

If you have a severe cough or a wheeze, the allergist may decide to postpone the skin tests until the symptom is less. This is because allergy skin tests may worsen your cough or wheeze.

I prefer not to perform allergy skin tests on a pregnant woman. First, the unlikely event of an allergic reaction during skin tests may complicate the pregnancy. Second, even if the allergy skin tests cause no problems, I do not like to start a mother's allergy treatment until after her baby's birth.

A child should be prepared for his visit to an allergist's office. It should be explained to him that he will have allergy skin tests and that these are performed with needles, but not that he will be given 20 or 40 injections. In particular, he should not be told that there will be no needles: such a child, when confronted by the nurse, feels cheated and even angry.

If the allergist hasn't told you, the appropriate question to ask is: "What am I allergic to?" rather than: "How many allergies do I have?"

You may feel weak after the tests. If this happens, rest in the allergist's office before you go into the street again. Also, it is better to stay quiet for an hour or so after allergy tests. If the arm tested is red, painful, or swollen, apply an icepack to reduce the swelling and take an allergy pill or antihistamine to reduce the redness and itching. Very rarely, allergy skin tests cause a serious anaphylactic reaction with a combination of symptoms such as choking or wheezing along with hives. If this happens, return immediately to the allergist's office or go to the nearest doctor or hospital emergency department. A delayed positive reaction may develop after 24 to 48 hours; such reactions, which are commonest after testing with mold antigens, are not very important in diagnosing an allergy. Extremely rare — in fact, an immunological curiosity — is the development of positive allergic reactions at the site of allergy skin tests done several months or years ago.

Before you leave the allergist's office, make sure you understand all the recommendations and instructions. Don't hesitate to ask questions. If you are going to have allergy injections, make sure you know exactly the procedure for ordering the allergy serum (it seems to vary so much from one doctor to another). If medication has been prescribed for you, be sure you know how to use it. In particular, if you will be using one of the many types of inhalers for the first time, it is very important that you understand how to use that particular type of inhaler. As you will probably need to repeat your prescription, have it filled at a pharmacy close to your home or work.

Allergy patients, particularly those on allergy injections, should be re-evaluated about every 2 years. The best time for your second appointment is about 1 month before completion of your second series of injections. Although most allergists seem to have a long waiting list, some amount of forethought will make this possible.

The best time to consult an allergist about hay fever is in the fall, so that treatment will be effective for next year's symptoms. A first visit to an allergist in the spring is too late for you to start treatment for that year's hay-fever season.

HISTORY OF SUSPECTED ALLERGY

If you think you have an allergy your best plan is to discuss it with your doctor rather than a friend or neighbor. And in order to get the most out of your visit to the doctor, get all your facts organized beforehand. List all your symptoms and put them in chronological order. You don't have to worry about medical terms; just describe your troubles in your own words. Then ask yourself the following questions and write in your answers: these constitute the historical facts your doctor will need to know.

Respiratory Allergy

1. Do your symptoms vary from one season to another? Do you have a good season or a bad season? Try to pinpoint the exact months. If you can't, try to relate your symptoms to holidays like Easter, school vacations, Labor Day, Halloween, Christmas and so on.
2. Are your symptoms influenced by the weather? Are they better in dry weather or humid weather?
3. Are you better indoors or outdoors?
4. How do you react in the company of animals? Have you had symptoms when in a barn or stable or at a horse show?
5. Have you noticed any association with foods?
6. Do your spells of cough and wheezing follow a cold or sore throat?
7. What is the color of your nasal secretions and the phlegm you cough up? Is it clear, or is it yellow, gray, or green?
8. Do you have a fever along with your symptoms?
9. Does exertion make your symptoms worse?
10. Do you cough more at night? Do you cough or sneeze more in certain places or during certain activities?
11. What kind of a furnace does your home have? Do you have a humidifier? Is there anything made of feathers or

wool in your bedroom? Is there a rug on the bedroom floor? Does anyone smoke in the bedroom? If your house has a basement, is it finished? Is there a workshop in your house? Are there any recreational activities in your house that would liberate dust or smells? How old is your house? Do you have a dog or cat or any other pets? Does your baby-sitter have pets? Did the previous tenants have any pets? Do you have a ski jacket or sleeping bag or quilt that contains feathers? Do you use a wool scarf?

12. Did you have eczema in infancy? Did you have any problems with foods in your infancy? Did you have many colds and upper respiratory infections before you started school? Did you have croup or asthma as a child? Have your tonsils been removed?

13. Is there any history of allergy in the family?

Skin Allergy

1. Does the rash come and go or is it there all the time? What are the factors that make it come or go?
2. On which parts of the body do you have the rash?
3. Is the rash itchy or red? Is it raised?
4. Do any parts of your body such as your lip or tongue swell?
5. Try to figure out whether the rash has any relationship to any clothing or footwear.
6. Make a list of all the cosmetics, toiletries, and household cleansers you use.
7. Do you come in contact with any unusual substances at home or at work or recreation?
8. Do you carry anything in your pockets?
9. Make a list of all metallic objects that come in contact with your body.
10. Does poison ivy grow in your backyard or nearby?
11. Make a list of all medications in your medicine chest.

157

Include all over-the-counter nonprescription medications that you have.

12. Is there any relationship between the rash and exertion and being overheated?
13. What is the influence of water or cold temperatures?
14. Are you an emotional person, and does your rash have anything to do with your emotional state?
15. What is the relationship between foods and your rash? If you have embarked on an elimination diet, what foods have you avoided?

Food Allergy

1. How soon after eating the suspected food do the symptoms develop?
2. Keep an accurate food diary of all foods and beverages.
3. Is there any rash, or redness or itching of your skin?
4. Did you have any trouble with foods as an infant?
5. If diarrhea is one of your symptoms, try to describe your stools. What color are they? Are they frothy? Do they float?
6. If you have been following some kind of an elimination diet, list all the foods you have been avoiding and for how long. Did you notice any improvement during this period of elimination?
7. Do you have any strong likes and dislikes for foods?

Insect Allergy

1. Are you talking about stinging insects (bee, wasp, yellowjacket and hornet) or biting insects (mosquito and flies)?
2. What kind of reactions do you get?
3. How soon after the bite do you get reactions? A few minutes? A few hours? A few days?
4. Do you get a generalized reaction or only at the site of the bite or sting?

5.   Do you have symptoms such as choking or wheezing or fainting?

Drug Allergy

1.   What are your exact symptoms?
2.   How soon after you took the drug did the symptoms appear?
3.   Did you have similar symptoms the last time you took this drug?
4.   Were you on any other medications at the time?

PHYSICAL EXAMINATION

After a good and detailed history comes the physical examination. This is no different from the examination of any other patient except that a few areas may be examined a little differently and more thoroughly.

The respiratory system begins with the nose. After observing the nose and nostrils and the surrounding skin, your doctor will look into your nose with a small flashlight-like device; this is called anterior rhinoscopy. He is looking at the structures of the nose and observing their color and the mucus inside. Next, he will examine your throat, paying special attention to the tonsils and the back of the throat. At this stage he might decide to do a posterior rhinoscopy to visualize your adenoids, the tonsil-like glands at the back of the nose. This examination is done with a little mirror. (Some doctors leave this examination to an ear, nose, and throat surgeon.) Next, the doctor will examine your eyes, ears, and neck. Finally, he will examine your chest. The doctor will observe the shape of the chest and the way it moves; he may tap it and listen to the sounds; and last, he will listen to your lungs through a stethoscope. While the doctor examines your chest you should breathe with your mouth open. He may ask you to cough, take a few deep breaths, exhale as much as you can or pant like a dog.

After your respiratory system the doctor will examine other systems of your body. And last, but not the least important, is the skin. The skin is the mirror of the body and reveals tell-tale signs of allergy.

ALLERGY TESTS

After the physical examination comes a series of tests. Most tests for allergy are simple and can be done in a doctor's office and certainly do not require a hospital stay.

1. A simple test to determine your total white-blood-cell count, with special emphasis on your eosinophil count, is often the first step. (Eosinophils are one type of white cells that increase in allergic conditions.)

2. Examination of the nasal mucus under the microscope is a relatively simple but valuable test.

3. Likewise, your sputum yields valuable information. Its color and consistency are very important. Sputum can also be cultured in a laboratory to find out what germs, if any, it contains.

4. X-ray films of the nose, sinuses, and chest add a lot of information, particularly if you have respiratory allergies.

5. Most people who have a definite or suspected allergy will need to have allergy tests. These are done not only to determine whether you have an allergy but also the degree of allergy. There are two types of allergy tests. The needle tests, which are done for inhalant, food, and insect allergy; and the patch tests, which are performed for contact allergy. Needle tests, again, are of two types: scratch tests and intradermal tests. For scratch tests, which are done on the forearm or further up the arm or on the back, scratches are made with a small screwdriver-like device; the results are read in about 20 minutes. Intradermal tests are performed with a very

superficial injection under the skin (similar to a T.B. test) higher on the arm or on the back, and the results are read in about 5 to 10 minutes. Some doctors do both kinds of tests and others do just one. A positive response consists in redness, a white swelling, and itching. Do not rub or scratch the area of the tests; an icepack will lessen the itching. Patch tests are done by putting a drop of the allergen on your skin and covering it with tape for about 24 to 48 hours. A positive reaction is manifested by redness and a swelling.

6. In certain circumstances your doctor may do what is called a provocation test. This is usually done in a hospital but you don't have to be admitted as an inpatient. For a provocation test you inhale the suspected allergen and its effects on your lungs are noted.

7. Pulmonary function studies are sometimes performed on patients who have asthma or other diseases of the lower respiratory tract. For these, you blow into tubes and other devices attached to machines and some of your blood constituents are measured.

THE ALLERGIST'S LINGO

Every profession and trade has its own lingo, and here are a few sentences an allergist does not particularly like hearing.

1. *"I have come to you because I don't think my previous allergist was very good."*
An allergist is an ordinary human being, like you and me, and may have a personality that doesn't suit every patient. Also, the allergist may have started you on the right treatment but your condition didn't improve because you didn't continue the treatment long enough.

2. *"Isn't everybody allergic to dust?"*
No, not everybody is allergic to dust, but most people

are intolerant of dust. Also, even though all dusts are irritants they are not necessarily allergens. It is house dust that concerns the allergist most.

3. *"There's a field behind my home, and that's where all the pollens seem to be coming from."*
It certainly doesn't help to have a field with tall grasses and weeds close by, but pollens may travel thousands of miles. You can be in a high-rise apartment in Ontario, inhaling grass pollen from Kentucky.

4. *"I knew I was allergic to wool because I can never wear a wool sweater."*
Itching caused by woolen clothing doesn't represent an allergy. This is primary skin irritation.

5. *"I have had my dog 5 years. Why am I allergic to it now?"*
It is because you have had the dog for 5 years that you are allergic to it now. The symptom-free period (the latent period) is the time your body has taken to develop enough antibodies to the specific allergen.

6. *"How many allergies do I have?"*
Allergy is not a numbers game. The proper question should be: "What am I allergic to?"

7. *"I think I have a sinus."*
Everyone has sinuses, including nasal ones. What you are trying to say is that you have symptoms of sinusitis. Also, do not use 'nose' and 'sinus' synonymously.

8. *"My own doctor told me I've got bronchitis. You tell me I have asthma. Who is right?"*
Both are right. The words bronchitis and asthma are quite often used interchangeably. Bronchitis refers to a condition characterized mainly by cough, and asthma to a condition characterized mainly by wheezing. However, bronchitics may also wheeze and asthmatics may also cough.

9. *"My child gets very frequent colds and I want him to start 'shots' for this."*

Unless these colds are caused by an underlying allergy, there is no such thing as 'shots for colds.'

10. *"My neighbor had 'shots' for poison ivy, and I want to get them too."*
There are no injections for poison ivy, and you would be better off talking about this to your doctor rather than your neighbor.

11. *"I discontinued my allergy injections for about 6 months and felt no worse, and therefore I feel I don't need them."*
Whether symptoms develop immediately or only some time after you discontinue allergy desensitization therapy depends on many factors.

12. *"I don't know why I'm here, but my mother asked me to get some allergy tests."*
History is the most important tool in diagnosing an allergic condition; without it, no amount of tests will help. If you cannot accompany your child to the allergist's office, please send a detailed written history with him or another family member who knows about the problem.

13. *"Shall I outgrow my allergies?"*
You may outgrow the symptoms of allergy, but you never outgrow the allergic state of your body.

14. *"I brought along some fibers from my rug and underpadding, and would like to be tested for that."*
It isn't possible to test you for your own rug or underpadding, or for that matter the dust in your home. Allergists carry standards that test for all the allergens likely to be present in an average home.

15. *"I know I'm not allergic to my hair dye, as I tried the skin test recommended by the manufacturers at home before applying the dye."*
The skin test referred to is a test for primary skin irritation, and not for contact allergy to hair dye. For contact allergy tests, the substances have to be kept in place on

163

the skin for about 48 hours.

16. *"My symptoms are much worse in the summer."*
This is not a very helpful statement. You must try to describe your allergy symptoms with reference to months rather than to seasons.

17. *"My last doctor gave me these little white pills and I felt much better on them."*
Many pills look alike. You should bring with you the containers that name the medications or have the name of the pharmacy where they were dispensed.

18. *"Although I'm on a refill of the same allergy serum, I felt much better on the last lot. Could there be something wrong with my new serum?"*
Allergic symptoms tend to vary, depending on many factors such as exposure to the allergens, infection in your respiratory system, your general health, your other anti-allergy medications such as antihistamines, and so on. These factors, rather than the new allergy serum, could be the source of your problem. In any case, there is no way to test an allergy serum once it is made. If you feel convinced there is something wrong with it — and I urge you to think many times before you come to this conclusion — you can ask for it to be remade. You will then have to re-start on the lowest dose and work upward — and you must bear in mind that, while these changes are taking place, your immunity lessens.

19. *Mother of two children in an allergist's office: "Both my children get too many colds and I have brought them for allergy tests."*
Although your children may have similar symptoms, it is more helpful if you describe each child's history individually and then mention any features that are common to both.

20. *"I would like to discontinue my allergy injections, because I have been having troublesome reactions."*

The paradox of this situation is that the patients who have troublesome reactions to allergy injections need their injections the most and experience the greatest improvement. Therefore, if you are one of those patients who have such reactions, the allergist is likely to advise you to continue the injections but with a reduced dosage or different schedule.

18

A GLOSSARY OF TERMS FOR THE ALLERGIC

FROM ADENOIDS TO ZOOPHILE

ADENOIDS Glandular tissue at the back of the nose.

ADRENALINE (EPINEPHRINE) A hormone which is produced by the body's adrenal glands and has a vital role in preserving life. Adrenalin is a trade name of the manufactured substance which may be life-saving in serious allergic reactions.

ALLERGEN A special group of antigens which are harmless to the majority of the population but may cause disease when allergy-prone individuals are exposed to them by inhalation, ingestion, or injection, or by contact with the skin.

ALLERGY BRACELET See Medical-alert Bracelet.

AMINOPHYLLINE A type of bronchodilator medication.

ANAPHYLACTIC REACTION Technically, certain types of allergic reactions like hay fever can be caused by an anaphylactic reaction. But the term usually is reserved for the serious acute allergic reaction that is characterized by urticaria, abdominal cramps, wheezing and shock. It can be caused by drugs, insect bites, and foods.

ANTIBODY Microscopic protein substances produced by the body in response to an antigen.

ANTIGEN A substance that can produce antibodies in the body and bind specifically with these antibodies.

ANTIHISTAMINE A medication which blocks the action of histamine that is released from cells in response to an allergic reaction.

ASTHMA A disease characterized by recurrent but reversible episodes of bronchospasms.

***BETA*-2 STIMULATOR** A type of bronchodilator medication.

BRONCHIOLITIS Inflammation of the bronchioles (small air passages that branch from the bronchi in your lungs), commonest in infants. It is accompanied by wheezing and may resemble asthma.

BRONCHITIS Inflammation of the bronchi (the larger air passages in your lungs).

167

BRONCHODILATOR A medication which opens bronchial passages that have become narrowed by respiratory disease.

BRONCHOSPASM A contraction of the muscles of the bronchi. It reduces the space within the air passages, thereby obstructing air flow.

CATARRH Excess mucus production secondary to inflammation of the mucous membrane in any part of the body, usually the nose and throat.

CHEMOPROPHYLAXIS Administration of antibiotics when infection is anticipated, to prevent development of the infection.

CONJUNCTIVITIS Inflammation of the lining of the eyes; causes redness, itching, tearing and a discharge.

CONTACT DERMATITIS The inflammation of the skin that develops as an allergic reaction to a substance you have come in contact with (e.g., metals, hair dye).

CORTISONE A very important hormone produced by the body's adrenal glands. Cortisone is available as a medication in the form of pills, liquid, inhalant and ointment.

CROMOLYN SODIUM A medication that prevents the release of histamine from the cells and, therefore, can prevent allergic symptoms relating to the respiratory tract.

CROUP (TRACHEOBRONCHITIS). Inflammation of the windpipe (trachea) and the larger air passages in the lungs.

DANDER Tiny scales from animal hair, feathers, and superficial layers of the skin, and saliva.

DERMATOGRAPHIA Literally, being able to write on the skin — without use of pen or pencil. Firm stroking with a blunt instrument produces a white raised urticarial weal with a red flare on either side.

DESENSITIZATION A process of building up your body's immunity by injecting minute amounts of antigens periodically over long periods. It is more correctly termed 'hyposensitization' as a patient cannot be completely desensitized, especially to substances he is exposed to constantly. See Sensitization.

ELIMINATION DIET Elimination of 1 or more foods for at least 3 weeks, followed by introduction of one of the foods in the fourth week, another some time later, and so on.

EOSINOPHIL A type of white blood cell. The number of eosinophils in the blood and nasal mucus may be increased in allergic diseases.

EPISTAXIS Nosebleed.

FOOD ADDITIVES Chemical substances that are added to foods to enhance flavor and appearance and as preservatives.

HAY FEVER A summer allergy with symptoms such as sneezing, nasal blocking and congestion, and so on.

HISTAMINE A chemical compound normally present in the body but which is produced in greatly increased amounts when an allergic reaction develops.

HIVES See Urticaria.

HOUSE DUST From the allergy point of view, house dust is not merely what you see on the tabletop or floor but a mixture of several organic substances in your home. Thus, house dust contains dust, human and animal hair and dander, cement, plaster, fibers from drapes, bedlinen, and carpets, contents of upholstery, construction material, and a microscopic insect (house-dust mite). See also Mite.

HUMIDIFIER An appliance that fans air through a water supply to increase the moisture content of air (humidity).

HYPOSENSITIZATION See Desensitization.

KAPOK A fiber used as padding in some clothing, toys, sleeping bags, upholstery, etc.

LARYNGOTRACHEOBRONCHITIS See Croup.

LATENT PERIOD The time between your first exposure to an antigen and the development of symptoms. It can vary from a few days to several years; therefore, you may experience no symptoms of allergy to a pet until several years after your acquired the animal, or no allergic reaction to a particular drug until you have had many doses.

MEDICAL-ALERT BRACELET A metal bracelet worn by patients who are allergic to insect stings or certain drugs or who have certain disorders that require specific treatment in an emergency.

MITE A microscopic insect that inhabits human and animal skin and feathers and is present in dark and dusty places like mattresses. House-dust mite is thought to be a major allergenic constituent of house dust.

MOLD A fungus or mildew that grows in damp places and on dead and decaying matter. It produces tiny particles (spores) that are a cause of allergic symptoms.

MUCOUS MEMBRANE The lining of certain passages in the body. It produces mucus. Specifically, the lining of the respiratory tract (from the tip of the nose down into the lungs).

MUCUS The sticky, normally clear watery substance produced by mucous membranes. Specifically, that which is produced in the respiratory tract.

NEBULIZER A device that delivers a spray of minute particles of medication into the respiratory system. Small nebulizers usually held in the hand are called inhalers.

PARASYMPATHETIC NERVE One of its functions is to make the bronchial muscles contract when it is stimulated. Together with the sympathetic nervous system, it contributes to the regulation of breathing.

PHARYNGITIS Inflammation of the pharynx (the area in the back of your mouth and nose).

PHOTOSENSITIVITY; PHOTOTOXICITY A condition in which exposure to sunlight causes problems such as rash, headaches, a burning sensation in the eyes and even vomiting.

PLANT DERMATITIS Inflammation of the skin, caused by an allergic reaction to plants or plant products.

POISON IVY A small three-leaved plant or shrub that grows wild throughout North America, including Mexico, and the West Indies. It can produce a troublesome form of contact dermatitis.

POLLEN The seeds of the flowers of plants and trees. To be able to affect humans, pollens must be microscopic and capable of being windborne. The allergic pollens are those of grasses, trees, and weeds. Pollens of other flowers are usually not allergenic.

POLLUTANT In relation to allergy, any airborne substance that irritates the respiratory tract.

POLYP Grape-like thickening of the mucous membrane (e.g., nasal polyp).

POSTNASAL DRIP Nasal secretions that drip down the back of the nose into the throat and upper air passages.

PULMONARY FUNCTION STUDIES Tests to measure the capacity and degree of function of your lungs, chiefly by measuring air volumes when you blow into certain machines and analysing the gases in your blood.

RESPIRATORY TRACT It starts at the entrance to your nostrils and runs through your nose to the back of your throat, down into your voice box (larynx) and windpipe (trachea), and then divides into 2 branches, 1 into each lung. These main branches are the large bronchi; they divide into smaller branches (the smaller bronchi), from which stem the bronchioles and, finally, the air sacs.

RESPIRATORY TREE The respiratory tract from larynx to air sacs.

SENSITIZATION A process that leads to the development of allergic symptoms in persons who are hypersensitive to the substance in question; for example, the first dose of penicillin you ever receive may sensitize your system to this antibiotic, so that the second or a later dose may cause an allergic reaction.

SEPTUM A piece of tissue that divides a cavity or area into two. The nasal septum is the structure that divides the nasal cavity into two nostrils.

SERUM (a) The liquid portion of blood. (b) In allergy, commonly used to describe the medication used to desensitize an allergic person; 'allergy serum' is the medication in the set of vials you receive from an allergist's office.

SINUS DRAINAGE A surgical procedure to drain infected material from sinuses.

SINUSITIS Inflammation of the air spaces around your nose.

SKIN TESTS Tests performed by an allergist on your skin. The principle on which the tests are based is as follows. A specific antigen is introduced into your system through your skin. If your body has a specific antibody to this antigen, it will react with it (produce an antigen–antibody reaction) and a small bump will appear at the site of the test.

STRIDOR The noisy breathing (during inspiration) typical of tracheobronchitis.

SYMPATHETIC NERVE Contributes to the regulation of breathing.

THEOPHYLLINE A type of bronchodilator medication.

TIC A 'nervous tic' is a neurotic habit, such as sniffing, throat-clearing, nail-biting and head-banging.

TONSIL A small gland on each side in your throat.

TRACHEOBRONCHITIS See Croup.

TUBERCULIN SYRINGE A special type of syringe used to administer allergy injections and perform skin tests. It has a capacity of 1 ml. and is graduated to read each 0.1 ml.

URTICARIA (HIVES) A skin reaction characterized by smooth, raised, itchy patches (weals) resembling mosquito bites, which are redder or paler than the surrounding skin.

VIAL A sealed glass bottle containing medication (e.g., allergy serum).

WHEEZING Musical, whistling, or rustling sounds, produced by the movement of air through narrowed air passages during expiration.

ZOOPHILE A lover of animals. Even if you are a zoophile, if a member of your family is allergic to dander you should not keep a furred or feathered pet.

ABOUT THE AUTHOR

Harsha Venilal Dehejia was born in Bombay, India, and graduated in Medicine from Bombay University in 1960. As a medical student he secured a gold medal in 6 out of 8 subjects in the medical curriculum, setting a new record for the University. Dr. Dehejia served his internship and 3 years' residency in internal medicine at the King Edward VII Memorial Hospital in Bombay. This was followed by graduate training in allergy and respiratory diseases in Cambridge, England, and almost 3 years at the famous Bellevue Hospital in New York, N.Y. During his graduate studies, Dr. H.V. Dehejia became a Member of the Royal Colleges of Physicians of both London and Glasgow by examination. He has further qualified as a Fellow of the Royal College of Physicians and Surgeons of Canada and has been elected a Fellow of the American College of Chest Physicians.

Dr. Dehejia lives in Ottawa, Ontario, where he practices as an allergist. His wife, Sudha, is a pediatrician. They have two boys, Vivek and Rajeev.

Dr. Dehejia is now working toward a degree in religion at Carleton University, Ottawa.

INDEX